POPULATION HEALTH MANAGEMENT

Strategies to Improve Outcomes

POPULATION HEALTH MANAGEMENT

Strategies to Improve Outcomes

by Ann Scheck McAlearney, Sc.D.

Health Administration Press, Chicago, Illinois
AUPHA Press, Washington, DC

AUPHA
HAP

Your board, staff, or clients may also benefit from this book's insight. For more information on quantity discounts, contact the Health Administration Press Marketing Manager at (312) 424-9470.

06   05   04   03   02   5   4   3   2   1

Library of Congress Cataloging-in-Publication Data

McAlearney, Ann Scheck.
    Population health management: strategies to improve outcomes / by Ann Scheck McAlearney.
      p. cm.
    Includes bibliographical references and index.
    ISBN 1-56793-187-1 (alk. paper)
    1. Managed care plans (Medical care)—Patients—Care.   2. Medical care—Needs assessment.   3. Health services accessibility.   I. Title.

  RA413 .M34 2002
  362.1'068—dc21   2002068550

The paper used in this publication meets the minimum requirements of American National Standard for Information Sciences—Permanence of Paper for Printed Library Materials, ANSI Z39.48-1984. ⊚™

Acquisitions editor: Marcy McKay; Project manager: Cami Cacciatore; Cover designer: Matt Avery

Health Administration Press
A division of the Foundation
  of the American College of
  Healthcare Executives
One North Franklin Street
Suite 1700
Chicago, IL 60606
(312) 424-2800

Association of University Programs
  in Health Administration
730 11th Street, NW
4th Floor
Washington, DC 20001
(202) 638-1448

To my sons, William and Brendan,
with so much love

TABLE OF CONTENTS

Part V Implementing Population Health Management Strategies

WEB SITE TABLE OF CONTENTS

To complement *Population Health Management: Strategies to Improve Outcomes,* a companion web site has been created at www.ache.org/pubs/mcalearney/start.cfm. This web site provides applied examples of the concepts described within the book, including population segmentation by age, geography, community, and employer; assessment tests and tools; and examples of cost containment strategies, disease management programs, injury prevention programs, and more.

In addition to enhancing your understanding of the concepts described in the text, this material offers additional resources for your research and self-study.

PREFACE

Why should we care about Population Health Management? The U.S. health-care system is less a system and more a fragmented and disorganized array of care providers, payers, and patients who are each challenged to look out for themselves in the chaos of the health services industry. The term population health management is used to describe different strategies that can be developed and implemented to improve health and the quality of care while also managing costs.

I decided to write this book to provide both students and practitioners with an understanding of strategies for health and care management for defined populations. Despite some semantic confusion about what population health management is or is not, from a managerial and organizational perspective, developing an understanding of strategies to improve the health and well-being of populations should be of great interest to both practitioners and students. When appropriately designed, targeted, and implemented, population health management strategies provide realistic opportunities to improve health while reducing costs.

While the field of population health management is developing and expanding rapidly, most available literature has tended to focus on individual health and medical management strategies. The goal of this book is to describe population health management strategies in a format that both students and practitioners can read and comprehend to inform their understanding about program development opportunities and activities. First, clarifying the perspective of the organization or payer developing such strategies helps frame program development decisions. Next, defining populations for health and care management interventions establishes parameters for effective health improvement approaches that will be appropriate for those defined populations. Then, targeting appropriate individuals within the defined populations for interventions sets the stage for different population health management strategies.

Five alternative strategies for population health management are presented to give each reader the opportunity to gain a better understanding of those programs and options in the healthcare field. In addition, the critical role of integration in population health management is emphasized. Chapters describing the importance of additional factors such as information technologies, care managers, physicians, and strategic management attempt to provide context and subject for population health management strategy development and implementation. Readers will be able to gain perspective about both the potential and appropriateness of individual population health management strategies and the implications of decisions they might make about more or less comprehensive approaches to population health management.

My perspective about population health management and my decision to write this book have been framed by my experience in both industry and academics. Working in a variety of health care settings—including an integrated delivery system, a managed care organization, academic medical centers, and community hospitals—has broadened my understanding of the different facets of the health services industry. Managing project teams, creating strategic and marketing plans, and directing development of a population health management program supported by integrated information technologies have given me practical experience and contributed to my understanding of the difficulties of program implementation and the realities of resource constraints and organizational politics. Information about alternative population health management strategies should assist practitioners in industry and facilitate the compare and contrast process that must inform management decisions about strategies to pursue.

As a faculty member teaching in the areas of strategy, leadership, and organizational management in healthcare, I am aware that specific strategies for population health management are often not introduced to management students. Nonetheless, when these students begin to work for various health services and consulting organizations, they are faced with projects such as developing disease management programs, implementing health and wellness programs, and trying to reduce the incidence of employee absence and disability. I have written this book to introduce some of these strategies and offer examples of how population health management strategies can work in practice.

The information collected in this book is organized to provide an overview of the different strategies and concepts I consider important in population health management. Although I have tried to be complete, the content is not exhaustive, and the rapidly changing nature of the healthcare industry ensures that some of this information will be out of date even as the book goes to press. It is my hope to provide readers with a thorough introduction to these subjects that may then stimulate them to pursue individual topics in greater depth.

Ultimately, the goal of such a book is to contribute to the field by increasing awareness of how we can provide better care and improve health across the whole population. Population health management strategies can contribute to this process and help management and health care practitioners who are trying to create an integrated system of care for all patients, across the care continuum.

ACKNOWLEDGMENTS

I want to thank the many people who have provided me with support and encouragement in the monumental process of writing this book. I am especially grateful to my colleague and friend, Steve Strasser, Ph.D., for his unswerving encouragement, prodding, and help with this process. Without his enthusiastic support and periodic working lunches, this book would likely remain unwritten.

My friend and former colleague, Roberta Suber, M.S.W., provided wonderful assistance as an objective reviewer and sounding board for the book. Her numerous suggestions, e-mailed articles, and friendly messages were invaluable. I also appreciate the insight and perspective provided by Debby Kweller, another friend and former colleague, who introduced me to the concept of disability management.

I offer sincere thanks to my external reviewer, Janet Buelow, Ph.D., for her incredibly thorough review and her help in providing concrete suggestions, conceptual clarity, and positive support. In addition, the kind reviews of David Kindig, M.D., Ph.D., and George Isham, M.D., were very encouraging.

Colleagues and students at the Ohio State University Graduate Program in Health Services Management and Policy were both supportive and enthusiastic about this process. Stephen Loebs, Ph.D., my department chair, provided wholehearted encouragement for writing this book. I want to especially thank Tracy Bryan for her prompt and friendly help in finding articles, collecting references, and helping to improve my productivity.

I would also like to thank my family and friends who helped support me in this process. My husband and best friend, John McAlearney, Ph.D., deserves profound thanks for his constant understanding during this process. He and my daughter, Fiona, have given me perspective and kept me happy along the way. My parents, Carol and Tim Scheck, my husband's parents, John and Pat McAlearney, and my sister and her husband, Gayle and Jason Northrop, were also wonderfully supportive.

Finally, I would like to express my sincere appreciation to Marcy McKay, Cami Cacciatore, and Audrey Kaufman of Health Administration Press for their dedication, support, and flexibility in this process. I am also profoundly grateful to Rob Fromberg, formerly of Health Administration Press, who was responsible for getting this book started.

OVERVIEW

INTRODUCTION

Strategies designed to improve the health and well-being of the public are increasing in both visibility and importance. *Population health management* is a term used to describe a variety of approaches developed to foster health and quality of care improvements while managing costs. Health services organizations faced with the challenge of managing financial risk for a defined population are challenged to find ways to more efficiently and effectively serve that population, and population health management strategies can help.

Strategies for health and care management that strive to improve quality as well as reduce the cost of medical care are appealing to payers, providers, and patients. As long as patient care needs are not subsumed by financial considerations, the potential for population health management programs to foster health improvements in a patient-centered and clinically responsive environment is undeniably attractive.

When managing health for a specific population, the characteristics of the defined population establish the parameters for what types of health improvement and management strategies will be appropriate. For instance, in a population with a high proportion of Native Americans, diabetes services may be more of a priority than in a population with more Caucasians. Similarly, an elderly population may need more attention to chronic disease management services while a younger population may be an appropriate target for maternal and child wellness programs or workplace injury reduction initiatives. Taking the characteristics of the target population into account when designing and implementing health management approaches is critical to ensure that such programs succeed in meeting appropriate and achievable health improvement goals.

Population health management strategies include many different initiatives. *Lifestyle management* approaches use the techniques of health behavior change in a health promotion or prevention context to improve individuals' health habits and reduce health risks. *Demand management* programs typically use remote patient management to direct individuals toward appropriate utilization of medical care services. *Disease management* strategies focus on a particular disease and attempt to provide medical and care management services related to the needs of patients with that condition. As another disease management model, *catastrophic care management* programs concentrate on providing the spectrum of services required by individuals who suffer from catastrophic illnesses or injuries that are typically defined by either condition or expensive claims. *Disability management* programs are usually developed from an employer perspective and try to bridge the gap between healthcare management and disability management to reduce lost worker productivity due to illness or injury. Finally, an *integrated population health management* model promotes comprehensive consideration of the health and well-being of each member of a population by coordinating different health and care management strategies. Each of these approaches is designed with specific goals and objectives in mind and makes patients' healthcare needs central to program development. By concentrating on the needs of individuals as they access the healthcare system or make decisions about their health behaviors, population health management programs hope to promote health and wellness among their defined populations and strive to manage healthcare costs without compromising the quality of healthcare provided.

Examples of population health management programs can be found in multiple settings. Employers may sponsor demand management programs while medical groups or health plans have interest in the potential of disease management to help improve health and reduce costs for their chronically ill patients. Disability management programs are being adopted by large employers, and catastrophic care management approaches may be offered through insurance carriers, employers, or dedicated vendor companies.

Population health management strategies are particularly common in managed care. A managed care organization (MCO) is typically trying to manage healthcare services for their defined population of members, keeping in mind both cost and quality of care. This defined MCO membership may be further segregated into subpopulations based on the managed care product lines that are offered. These subpopulations may include a commercial population, a Medicare population, or a Medicaid population, depending on the membership served. Developing health management strategies that address the needs of its membership can help both patients and the MCO by focusing on health improvements and trying to manage the costs of medical care.

The need to focus on service and health improvements for defined populations is increasingly important from both payer and provider perspectives. Methods to identify and care for segments of the population that are utilizers of health services leverage the capabilities of information technologies to obtain timely information about individuals and their care progress. New provider types such as care managers are working to respond to patient care and care coordination needs. Population health management programs with the potential to integrate quality improvement goals with cost-saving goals can have a tremendous impact on care delivery and outcomes.

A Case for Population Health Management

Shifting demographics, the tremendous burden of chronic illness and disability, and the problem of fragmentation in the U.S. healthcare system are three major factors increasing the visibility and need for population health management solutions. The challenges presented by these issues can be addressed by population health management solutions as health services organizations attempt to focus on both service and health improvements.

Demographics

One of the reasons population health management is increasing in importance is the shifting demographics of the U.S. population. By 2000, almost 13 percent of the U.S. population, or 35 million individuals, were age 65 or older. This proportion has increased over ten-fold since 1900 when persons over 65 represented only 4 percent of the U.S. population. By 2030, one in five Americans are projected to be age 65 or older as this population segment doubles to 70 million persons. Individuals age 85 and older represent the fastest growing older population segment. While 4 million persons, or 2 percent of the U.S. population, were estimated to be age 85 and older in 2000, this number is projected to increase by 5 percent to 19 million individuals by 2050 (Federal 2000).

With the average age of the population increasing and life expectancies extending as well, users of medical care services will be older. These shifts in age are also associated with an increase in the number of persons suffering from chronic conditions. Elderly persons experience a greater proportion of chronic illnesses, with 47 percent of older adults suffering from arthritis, 37 percent from hypertension, 29 percent from heart disease, and 17 percent from orthopedic impairments (Haber 1994). Elderly persons tend to need more medical care services than younger persons, and the population segment age 85 and older tends to be in the poorest health, requiring the most services among the elderly population overall (Federal 2000). Chronic illnesses and poor health are clearly associated with a greater need for medical care services, and these services can be expensive, difficult to access, and largely uncoordinated.

Additional shifts in U.S. demographics indicate increasing proportions of women, minorities, and poor people who will need healthcare services in most communities. Because population health management programs must begin by defining target populations, these shifting demographics will undoubtedly have implications for program development. Among the elderly, women were estimated to represent 58 percent of the U.S. population age 65 and over in 2000, and 70 percent of the age 85 and over population (Federal 2000). Disease management programs, for example, can focus on conditions that specifically target women or particular minority groups. A women's wellness program may be designed to serve a population of women past childbearing age who are starting to deal with menopause. Similarly, a disease management program that targets diabetes may be a priority program development area for a population with more low-income and minority persons for which uncontrolled diabetes and diabetes-related morbidity have been shown to be major problems (U.S. Department of Health and Human Services 1999). Keeping these demographic issues in mind helps establish a framework for population health management approaches as they are implemented for individuals.

Chronic Disease and Disability

Chronic illness is a major problem in the United States where, as of 2000, almost half of all Americans were found to be living with some form of chronic disease. Among these 125 million individuals, around 60 million have multiple chronic conditions, and over 3 million live with 5 chronic conditions (Partnership for Solutions 2001). According to the Institute for Health and Aging (1996), approximately 40 million persons experience definite limitations in their activities of daily living because of their chronic conditions.

Unfortunately, the numbers of disabilities and limitations due to chronic conditions are on the rise. Since 1991, the proportion of individuals who report experiencing a limitation in a major activity because of a chronic condition has been increasing for all population groups (U.S. Department of Health and Human Services 1999). The number of Americans projected to have at least one chronic condition by 2020 is almost 157 million individuals (Partnership for Solutions 2001).

Considering expenses, the cost of chronic illness is staggering. In fact, the Institute for Health and Aging of the University of California at San Francisco estimated that the medical care costs for people with chronic diseases were responsible for over 60 percent of U.S. medical care costs (The Robert Wood Johnson Foundation 1996). Partnership for Solutions is an initiative led by Johns Hopkins University and The Robert Wood Johnson Foundation designed to improve care and the quality of life for Americans with chronic health conditions. They estimate that the direct medical costs associated with chronic conditions reached $510 billion by 2000, and they project that these costs will increase to $1.07 trillion by 2020 (Partnership for Solutions 2001). Annual out-of-pocket medical care costs for individuals with chronic conditions are estimated to be about $369, almost double those of persons without such conditions. Total medical expenditures for those with chronic conditions are over five times greater than for healthy individuals, at $6,032 per year compared to $1,105 per year (Partnership for Solutions 2001).

The cost of disability attributable to chronic conditions in the United States is also overwhelming. For employers alone, the cost of lost productivity from both illness and injury represents 74 percent of their total employee benefit costs (Integrated Benefits Institute 2001). Individuals who have functional limitations or disabilities in addition to chronic conditions are estimated to have medical expenditures over twice as high as those with chronic conditions alone. These expenses are calculated as $10,908 per year for those with a disability in addition to a chronic condition, and $16,245 per year for those with functional limitations as well as a chronic condition (Partnership for Solutions 2001).

Another major issue associated with chronic diseases is the problems that may result from untreated primary illnesses (Suber 2001). If such conditions are not managed well, many chronic diseases will result in secondary conditions (Pope and Tarlow 1991) caused by the existing condition. As an example, diabetes is a chronic disease that can result in multiple disabling complications including heart disease, stroke, blindness, and amputations. Analysis of data from 1997 showed that over half of the 67,000 limb amputations in the United States could have been prevented if diabetics had managed their chronic illness better through routine foot exams ("Get a Foothold" 1998).

Given the high prevalence of and cost associated with chronic conditions in the United States, it would make sense that care provision for these illnesses would be a focus. However, the U.S. medical care system has tended to focus on acute care services. Even when treatment for acute exacerbations of chronic illnesses is provided, such care is rarely coordinated with other services that a patient is receiving or needs. Most care for chronic conditions is disorganized and difficult to obtain, with many services provided that are inappropriate or duplicative (Robert Wood Johnson Foundation 1996).

When properly designed and implemented, population health management programs can help to improve the care of persons with chronic conditions by both improving patient health and well-being and reducing medical care costs. In fact, the goal of chronic care is not necessarily to cure patients but to help individuals maintain their independence and functionality at high levels (Robert Wood Johnson Foundation 1996). By defining target populations and then designing health management programs to address the care requirements for individuals in those populations, comprehensive programs can be effectively introduced into an otherwise disjointed system of care.

Fragmentation

Organization and delivery of medical care services in the United States is extremely fragmented. Due in large part to the foundations of the medical care system as a decentralized cottage industry that has not emphasized coordination or continuity of care (Starr 1982), the present healthcare system is very disorganized. In general, the health of the U.S. population as a whole has not improved as rapidly as might have been predicted based on advances in medical care and technology (U.S. Department of Health and Human Services 1990). Instead, indicators of health leave much room for system improvement, whether measured on the basis of life expectancy, childhood mortality, health-adjusted life expectancy (Kindig 1998), or disability-adjusted life expectancy (World Health Organization 2000).

Fragmentation is problematic in multiple levels of the healthcare system, including patient care, provider, organization, financing, and overall health policy (Shortell et al. 1996). Multiple providers involved in patient care, complex organizational and financial structures, and health policy issues such as access, insurance coverage, costs, and quality all complicate healthcare management and delivery (McAlearney 2002). This uncoordinated service provision presents a major opportunity for population health management programs that can be designed to organize and integrate services across institutions, among providers, and along the continuum of care.

Population Health Management Framework

Population health management strategies fit into an overall framework for population health management that is illustrated in Figure 1. As shown in this figure, the first step in population health management is to target the specific program. This targeting process involves determining the perspective of the program and the concerns of the sponsoring organization, defining the population that will be managed, developing approaches to target individuals for health and care management strategies, and classifying those individuals for population health management interventions.

After targeting populations and individuals within those populations for health management interventions, the next stage in this process is to determine the appropriate strategies for population health management. In this text, five strategic options are described: lifestyle management, demand management, disease management, catastrophic care management, and disability management. Depending on the strategy selected, implementation issues such as design, development, and management of the program will vary. Issues around planning and organization, staffing, physician relations, organizational change, program evaluation, and strategic control of the process are all important.

Critical issues in program design, development, and implementation must be resolved to ensure that a population health management program is effective. Areas such as incentive alignment, program focus, and physician involvement should all be addressed to maximize the likelihood of program success. Program staff must be recruited and trained, and investments must be made in appropriate information technologies.

Clearly, given the debilitating fragmentation and lack of coordination in the U.S. healthcare system, better management of population health is needed. Population health management strategies provide an opportunity to improve the delivery and outcomes of medical care in the context of the existing U.S. healthcare system.

Organization and Summary

Parts of the book are organized to follow the framework for population health management shown in Figure 1. This first part describes population health management in general and gives appropriate definitions. Chapter 2 follows with a general overview of the concept of population health management. Part II sets the stage for developing population health management strategies by describing the processes needed to target population health management programs. Chapter 3 discusses the importance of defining the perspective of population health management programs and defining specific populations for management. Chapter 4 continues this discussion of preparing for population health management by discussing the importance of targeting and stratifying individuals for population health management interventions.

Part III of the text presents five specific strategies for population health management. Lifestyle management is discussed first in Chapter 5 as a consumer-focused approach to health management. Chapter 6 presents demand management as a more guided approach to health management. Next, disease management is described in Chapter 7, with an emphasis on disease management for chronic conditions. Chapter 8 follows with a discussion of catastrophic care management and is an extension of the disease management discussion. This health management approach moves beyond chronic illness management to consider catastrophic illnesses and injuries that are less predictable in occurrence and have more variation in treatment. The final chapter of this section, Chapter 9, presents disability management. While this topic is not often discussed in the context of health management, disability management is an extremely important component of the population health management equation from the perspective of employers. Including this discussion helps expand consideration of population health management approaches from the perspectives of multiple payers and participants.

Part IV of the book describes the importance of integrating population health management strategies. This integrated population health management approach is presented in Chapter 10. Next, Part V discusses some of the important aspects of implementing population health management strategies. Chapter 11 provides a discussion about strategic program management in program development and implementation. Care managers and their pivotal role are discussed in Chapter 12, and Chapter 13 describes the important roles of physicians in population health management. Chapter 14 discusses the value of incorporating information technologies in any population health management program. Finally, Chapter 15 concludes the book with a discussion of how to leverage opportunities in population health management through effective management and health services research.

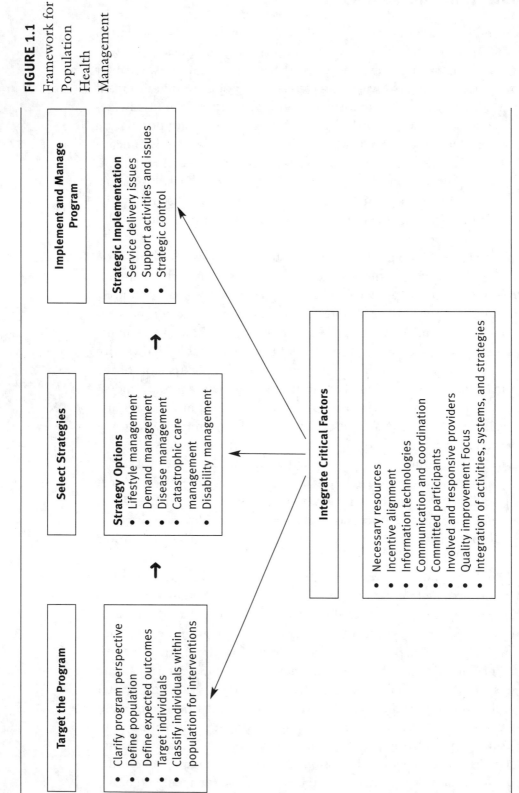

FIGURE 1.1
Framework for Population Health Management

Target the Program

- Clarify program perspective
- Define population
- Define expected outcomes
- Target individuals
- Classify individuals within population for interventions

Select Strategies

Strategy Options
- Lifestyle management
- Demand management
- Disease management
- Catastrophic care management
- Disability management

Implement and Manage Program

Strategic Implementation
- Service delivery issues
- Support activities and issues
- Strategic control

Integrate Critical Factors

- Necessary resources
- Incentive alignment
- Information technologies
- Communication and coordination
- Committed participants
- Involved and responsive providers
- Quality improvement Focus
- Integration of activities, systems, and strategies

SOURCE: Adapted from Janet Buelow. 2002. Personal communication, February.

REFERENCES

Federal Interagency Forum on Aging-Related Statistics. 2000. *Older Americans 2000: Key Indicators of Well-Being.* Washington, DC: Federal Interagency Forum on Aging-Related Statistics, U.S. Government Printing Office.

"Get a Foothold on the Cost of Diabetes Complications." 1998. *Healthcare Demand and Disease Management* 4 (5): 65–69.

Haber, D. 1994. *Health Promotion and Aging.* New York: Springer Publishing Company.

Integrated Benefits Institute. 2001. [Online article or information; retrieved 3/14/01.] http://www.ibiweb.org/breaking-news/index.shtml.

Kindig, D. A. 1998. "Purchasing Population Health: Aligning Financial Incentives to Improve Health Outcomes." *Health Services Research* 33 (2): 223–42.

McAlearney, A. S. 2002. "Population Health Management in Theory and Practice." In *Advances in Health Care Management* (Volume 3), edited by G. T. Savage, J. Blair, and M. Fottler. New York: JAI Press/Elsevier Science, Ltd.

Partnership for Solutions. 2001. *Prevalence and Cost of Chronic Conditions.* Baltimore, MD: Partnership for Solutions. [Online article or information; retrieved 2/6/02.] http://www.chronicnet.org/statistics/issue_briefs. htm; http://www.chronicnet.org/statistics/prevalence.htm.

Pope, A. M., and A. R. Tarlow. 1991. *Disability in America: Toward a National Agenda for Prevention.* Washington, DC: National Academy Press.

Shortell, S. M., R. R. Gillies, and D. A. Anderson. 1996. *Remaking Health Care in America: Building Organized Delivery Systems.* San Francisco: Jossey-Bass Publishers.

Starr, P. 1982. *The Social Transformation of American Medicine.* New York: Basic Books.

Suber, R. M. 2001. "Total Health Management: Prevention and Management of Chronic Disease." In *The Continuum of Long-Term Care,* edited by C. Evashwick. Albany, NY: Delmar Publishers.

The Robert Wood Johnson Foundation. 1996. *Chronic Care in America: A 21st Century Challenge.* Princeton, NJ: The Robert Wood Johnson Foundation.

U.S. Department of Health and Human Services. 1990. *Healthy People 2000: National Health Promotion and Disease Prevention Objectives.* Publication No. (PHS) 91-50213. Washington, DC: U.S. Department of Health and Human Services.

U.S. Department of Health and Human Services. *Healthy People 2000 Review 1998–99.* 1999. Publication No. (PHS) 96-1256. Washington, DC: U.S. Department of Health and Human Services.

World Health Organization. 2000. *World Health Report.* Geneva, Switzerland: World Health Organization. [Online article or information; retrieved 3/14/01.] http://www.who.int/whr/2000/en/report.htm.

POPULATION HEALTH MANAGEMENT

A book about population health management must begin by clarifying what is meant by population health management. This chapter poses the following four questions:

1. *What* is to be managed in population health management?
2. *Who* is to be managed?
3. *Where* can population health management occur?
4. *Why* does population health need to be managed?

Answers to these four questions will help establish a context for individual population health management strategies, as well build support for their practical importance in the U.S. healthcare system. The remainder of the book will then attempt to explain *how* population health management can occur.

What Is to Be Managed?

Considering the issue of population health management, one of the first questions that arises is what is meant by *health*? Definitions of health and well-being have been put forth by a number of entities. Best known is the definition used by the World Health Organization (WHO) that states, "Health is a state of complete physical, mental, and social well-being and not merely the absence of disease or infirmity" (WHO 1948). This definition is effective in the context of population health as well, because the goals of preventing disease, improving well-being, and promoting healthy behaviors are all integral parts of population health management.

Another definitional issue surrounds the concept of *management*. When used in the context of a business, management is defined as an operational process. Management is geared towards achieving the objectives of that business, whether those objectives are focused on maximizing revenues, value to shareholders, or benefit to society. In the context of healthcare, management can again be viewed as an operational process designed to achieve specific objectives. However, within the realm of health services, the objectives of healthcare management are geared towards attaining, maximizing, or improving health, as health is defined above. In population health management, the objective of management is to maximize the health of a population.

This leads to the third part of the term population health management: *population*. Why is it important to consider health management within a population separate from health management in general? The goal of managing health within a defined population has become a critical issue for many. Whether the population specified is that of a health plan's membership, a hospital's patients, an employer's employees, or a community's citizens, the issue of describing that population and determining the needs of individuals as members of that group is central. By specifying a population group, a health management program can be initiated that responds to the needs of that group. This perspective helps establish boundaries for a health management program by defining a population of concern.

The broadest definitions of populations are, of course, national or global. Considering the goals of the World Health Organization, the global population is the population of interest, and programs are designed to help improve the health and well-being of the world's residents. However, beyond acknowledging the health needs of the world's population, even WHO effectively defines and segments populations when it designs specific health programs. An initiative to control the spread of tuberculosis in less developed countries will not be targeted to reach residents in U.S. suburbs. Similarly, messages about reducing the spread of HIV and AIDS may be substantially different depending on whether the target audience consists of intravenous drug users in urban areas or sex workers in less developed countries. Defining a population for a health management program allows such initiatives to concentrate resources and tailor messages in ways that will be most effective for that population.

Multiple forces influence health. In addition to the medical care system, nonmedical factors such as socioeconomic status (Adler et al. 1994), education (Pappas et al. 1993), income (Kaplan et al. 1996), individual behaviors (McGinnis and Foege 1993), social support, genetics, and the physical environment can all affect individual health (Kindig 1998). Figure 2.1 illustrates how these various factors can affect both personal outcomes, including clinical health and functional status, and population health outcomes, such as health-adjusted life expectancy (Kindig 1998; 1997), as they are moderated by the roles played by intervening agents including healthcare organizations, care providers, and the government. (See 2.1 "Measuring Population Health Outcomes" at www.ache.org/pubs/mcalearney/start.cfm.)

For the United States, the management and improvement of health is a major financial, political, and social issue. The Healthy People initiative was designed as a national, cooperative effort by the government, in partnership with both voluntary and professional organizations, to try to improve the health of Americans. Objectives for health were established and progress toward the achievement of those objectives is measured (Suber 2001). Healthy People 2000 included three broad goals covering 300

FIGURE 2.1
Influencing
Health

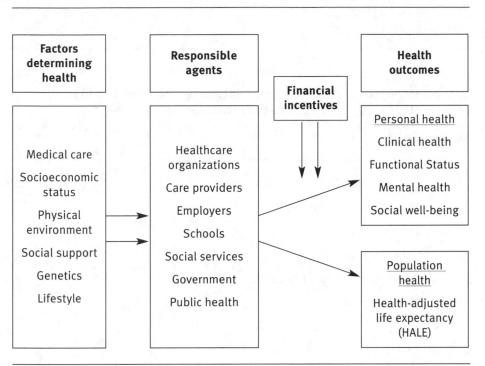

SOURCE: Kindig, D. A. 1998. "Purchasing Population Health: Aligning Financial Incentives to Improve Health Outcomes." *Health Services Research* 33 (2): 223–42.

specific objectives across 22 priority health areas: 1) to increase the span of healthy life; 2) to reduce health disparities; and 3) to achieve access to preventive services (U.S. Department of Health and Human Services 1990).

Prevention and health promotion goals for the U.S. were updated as 2000 approached, and Healthy People 2010 now includes 467 objectives covering 28 focus areas. Main goals were also refined for Healthy People 2010 and these are: (1) to increase quality and years of healthy life; and (2) to eliminate health disparities, including disparities due to race, ethnicity, gender, income, and insurance status. In addition to health goals and objectives, 10 leading health indicators were developed to focus the attention of the nation on needed health promotion and disease prevention strategies. These health indicators for 2010 are: (1) physical activity; (2) overweight and obesity; (3) tobacco use; (4) substance abuse; (5) responsible sexual behavior; (6) mental health; (7) injury and violence; (8) environmental quality; (9) immunization; and (10) access to healthcare (Centers for Disease Control and Prevention 2001). Health goals and health indicators for 2010 are displayed in Table 2.1. Healthy People 2010 now provides perspective about the many facets of health and well-being that can be managed and improved for Americans using population health management strategies.

TABLE 2.1

National
Health Goals
and Health
Indicators
for 2010

Health Goals

| 1. | To increase quality and years of healthy life |
| 2. | To eliminate health disparities, including disparities due to race, ethnicity, gender, income, and insurance status |

Health Indicators

1)	Physical activity
2)	Overweight and obesity
3)	Tobacco use
4)	Substance abuse
5)	Responsible sexual behavior
6)	Mental health
7)	Injury and violence
8)	Environmental quality
9)	Immunization
10)	Access to healthcare

SOURCE: Centers for Disease Control and Prevention. 2001. *Healthy People 2010*. Washington DC: National Center for Health Statistics.

Who Is to Be Managed?

In addition to the issue of what will be managed is the consideration of who will be managed in a population health framework. Indeed, defining a particular population whose health is to be managed is the first step in determining how to manage that population's health. As described above, populations can be defined in many different ways, and individuals may be members of different population groups. Membership in these different population groups will affect individuals as programs are designed and implemented to help them manage their own health, as well as that of their peers within the population group.

As an example, a 50-year-old woman employed by a major bank in a metropolitan area who has health insurance can be considered a member of three distinct population subgroups: she is an employee of the bank, a citizen of that community, and a member of the particular health insurance plan that provides her coverage. Each of these three populations has a vested interest in managing her health, both for her own benefit and the benefit of these groups (the bank, the community, the health plan) that have a social and/or financial interest in her health and well-being.

First, this woman's employer wants her to remain healthy so that she will be a productive employee, miss few days of work, and perform her job on a regular basis. To that end, the employer may have a health promotion program in place to encourage her to quit smoking, maintain a healthy weight, and reduce stress. The employer may also offer an Employee Assistance Program (EAP) designed to help her if she has any personal problems such as grief, alcohol dependence, or legal concerns that might interfere with her ability to perform her job.

As a member of the second population group, her community, this woman may be part of community-wide projects that have been developed to improve her individual health and personal well-being. Her community may participate in a project designed to facilitate data sharing among healthcare institutions throughout the city. For example, medical record data may be shared among healthcare facilities making it easier for all healthcare providers to offer coordinated care to individual patients regardless of practice setting. Similarly, there may be a statewide initiative in place to reduce smoking by making smoking illegal in public places. Her membership in this community population enables her to take advantage of such health improvement initiatives, either knowingly or unwittingly, as they affect her daily life.

Finally, as an insured member of a health plan, the woman is a member of a third population whose specific interest is also to oversee and manage her health. A health plan may offer a demand management program designed to support health plan members as they make decisions about appropriate healthcare utilization. Furthermore, if this woman has a chronic disease such as diabetes, she may be enrolled in a disease management program that has been developed to help her manage her condition and avoid costly and dangerous complications of the disease. Other programs such as reminders to get a mammogram or an initiative to encourage her to get an annual immunization against influenza may also be in place to help this woman and others like her receive preventive services on an appropriate schedule.

A population health management framework relies upon the notion of defining a population in order to assess the health and medical care needs of the individuals of concern. Chapter 3 provides an extended discussion of this topic to clarify the issues raised by population definition.

Where Can Management Happen?

Given the variety of population health management programs that can be developed, such strategies are appropriate in a number of settings. Employers, communities, and health plans all provide settings in which programs can be implemented to address the needs of distinct populations. Which programs are selected depends on the characteristics of the population to be managed, as well as how easily the individuals in that population can be reached and influenced to change their health behaviors. The federal government, for example, may be interested in having all its citizens eat five servings of fruits and vegetables each day, but it can do little to mandate this personal health behavior. Instead, a state-level initiative may concentrate on those health issues that it can legislate, such as developing mandatory seatbelt and helmet laws, enforcing mandatory speed limits, and prohibiting smoking in public places. Similarly, a community-wide initiative may be developed to publicize quality and accreditation information about healthcare facilities and adult day care centers to inform local citizens about such facilities. Entities with this broad level of concern but limited control over individual behaviors may need to concentrate health management initiatives on particular subpopulations or on strategies such as education and legislation appropriate for the entire population.

Employer-level initiatives, in contrast to governmental initiatives, are often developed to take advantage of the employer's access to the employee population. This immediate access may also be associated with the potential ability of an employer to have more influence over employees' lives than a state or community may have. An employer concerned about getting employees to quit smoking may prohibit smoking on its premises, offer a financial incentive in health insurance premiums for nonsmokers, and provide complete insurance coverage for smoking cessation programs and nicotine patches to encourage all employees to quit. Beyond smoking cessation, lifestyle management programs may be put in place that are designed to increase employee knowledge about healthy behaviors by providing health information and incentives such as discounted health club memberships. Depending on the needs of the employee population, employers may contract with health plans or independent businesses to provide specific population health management services that meet both employee needs and their own needs as employers try to maintain a productive workforce and contain their healthcare premium costs.

Population health management initiatives are also developed at the level of institutions such as health insurance plans and healthcare facilities. Demand management and disease management programs may be offered at the health plan level to facilitate self-care management and appropriate utilization. Comprehensive strategies designed to coordinate care or help with disease management and catastrophic care management are increasingly available within both the health plan setting and at the individual provider level for those providers who have the incentives to manage and improve patients' health.

Considering the needs of the target population as well as the organization developing or paying for the health management program will help ensure that programs are designed and implemented in settings appropriate to achieve desired outcomes. As an example, for a demand management programs where remote care management is the primary form of patient contact, geographic location is less important than for programs such as disease management or catastrophic care management initiatives that incorporate face-to-face contacts with their participants. Structuring programs to focus specifically on attaining defined outcomes such as clinical improvements, functional status improvements, or less time lost from work will also help inform the *where* of the program location decision by establishing parameters for participant contact and expected provider communications.

Why Does Population Health Need to Be Managed?

The issue of why population health needs to be managed involves the concept of scarce resources. Healthcare resources are finite, and healthcare expenditures continue to increase. The United States spent $1.3 trillion in national healthcare expenditures in 2000, a 6.9 percent increase over 1999 (Levit et al. 2002; CMS 2002). With approximately 14 percent of the United States' gross domestic product (GDP) dedicated to healthcare spending, the U.S. ranks first among all nations in health expenditures.

Average health spending per person in the United States was $4,637 in 2000 (Levit et al. 2002). However, this expenditure level does not guarantee health for all Americans. Data from a recent comparison of 13 countries showed that the United States actually ranks an average of 12th on a variety of health indicators, including ranking 11th in life expectancy for females at age 1, and 12th for males at age 1 (Starfield 2000). Using different indicators of health such as disability-adjusted life expectancy, child survival to age 5, and other metrics, the World Health Organization ranked the United States as 15th among 25 industrialized countries in 2000 (World Health Organization 2000).

Managing the health of a defined population must include the health policy considerations of access, cost, and quality. First, in defining the population served, access to healthcare services is a major issue, and access problems and disparities should be addressed as much as possible. Similarly, the cost of providing healthcare services to support that population must be taken into consideration. Depending on the organization or government funding or providing services, the cost of including population health management services must also be accounted for within a program budget. Limits on the available budget may determine what type of strategies for population health management are feasible for that population. Finally, the issue of the quality of healthcare services must also be taken into account. The actual quality of healthcare services must be monitored, health outcomes must be tracked, and the quality of healthcare management services must be assessed. By keeping these health policy issues in the forefront of considerations about population health management programs, the likelihood of improvements in health for individual participants and financial health for payers will be increased.

Access

Access to healthcare and health insurance is not well-established in the United States. In fact, the United States is the only developed country that does not provide guaranteed insurance coverage for all citizens and thereby does not ensure access to health services. By the end of the twentieth century, over 42 million Americans lacked health insurance, or 16 percent of the U.S. population (U.S. Census Bureau 2000). For children, the statistics are just as grim; studies revealed 11 million uninsured children in 1996, 90 percent of whom lived in households with at least one working adult.

The lack of universal coverage in the United States fundamentally contributes to the problem of controlling healthcare costs because poor, sick, and uninsured people have considerable difficulty seeking and receiving preventive services. In addition, the fragmented healthcare financing system requires that a safety net remain in place for those poor and uninsured. This partial solution is expensive and creates further problems by encouraging cost shifting for healthcare services as providers subsidize un-reimbursed care with fees obtained from insured patients (Anderson et al. 1996).

From a population health management perspective, access is a critical issue. In general, access to most health management programs is associated with some sort of private or government insurance coverage. Health plans like health maintenance organizations (HMOs) may offer options such as disease management programs to their members, while employers contract with demand management companies to help improve their employees' health and wellness. State Medicaid programs consider disease management programs to help manage their chronic illness costs, and hospitals, insurance companies, and provider groups work with catastrophic care management programs to limit their losses from catastrophic medical events.

Traditionally, employers have shared health insurance premiums with their employees through employee benefit packages so that employees are not fully responsible for the actual costs of their insurance or their medical care. However, when firms elect not to provide health insurance coverage or when individuals are unemployed, health insurance coverage may be prohibitively expensive for individual purchase. Government insurance coverage options such as Medicaid and Medicare are available to members of certain populations of individuals; however, if disability, income, or age criteria are not met, these individuals can remain uninsured.

Individuals who lack health insurance coverage do not have access to the health and wellness benefits of many population health management programs. Instead of being members of defined population groups targeted for health management, uninsured adults and children face a myriad of potential health and disability problems. Being uninsured is often associated with poorer health status, lack of a usual source of care, and abysmal rates for preventive health screenings such as immunizations, pap smears, and mammograms. Although in an ideal world this disenfranchised group should be a perfect target for population health management, their lack of insurance means that no sponsor exists to pay for the program, regardless of the potential benefits.

Optimally, while access to health management services is usually tied to health insurance coverage, opportunities may exist to leverage the value of such programs in ways that support uninsured and underinsured individuals. Programs that succeed in lowering medical care costs for covered individuals may be able to divert saved resources to provide care for the underserved. Health management programs that save providers time may succeed in supporting initiatives to use that time to provide services to uninsured or underinsured individuals in need of care but unable to pay. More specifically, developing a disease management program under the auspices of a particular insurance plan but extending the reach of the program to individuals who are uninsured or underinsured could be effective. (See 2.2 "Health Reform to Expand Access to Care Benefits from Population Health Management at www.ache.org/pubs/mcalearney/start. cfm.)

For the employer dedicated to community improvement and to supporting employees in their community service efforts, health management programs may present another opportunity to provide such service. Offering access to a lifestyle management or demand management program for members of an underserved community may be a valuable contribution to that community. For health plans and vendors providing health management services, dedicating a portion of company proceeds or time to providing services to underserved individuals is a very effective way of showing support for the community and for the goals of health improvement. Applying creativity in the development and implementation of health management initiatives can help promote the values of access to care and health services in the broader population as more individuals are included in defined population groups that can benefit from health management services.

Cost

As noted above, healthcare spending in the United States far exceeds expenditures in all other developed countries. Yet even at this expenditure level, medical care services are unaffordable for many Americans. Increases in technology and expertise have led to amazing success in the clinical treatment of disease. New technologies have made early diagnosis possible, and new treatments have extended as far as permitting surgical intervention on fetuses in the womb, and the identification and treatment of genetic anomalies. However, even with increased technology and high costs, health indicators for Americans are not as good as for residents of many other countries.

Containing healthcare costs has been a major goal of U.S. healthcare reform efforts. As described by Thomas Rice, conceptually, there are two categories of cost containment methods: methods based on fee-for-service reimbursement, and methods based on capitation (Anderson et al. 1996). Because population health management programs can be applied in either financial environment, attempts to contain costs under both systems will be briefly discussed. The importance of the concept of financial risk is also described, as is the overall perspective of using population health management strategies to reduce healthcare costs.

Fee-for-Service Systems

Cost containment strategies based on fee-for-service fall into three groups: price controls, volume controls, and expenditure controls (Rice 1996). Among these groups, the literature shows many examples of cost containment strategies including diagnosis-related groups and hospital rate-setting programs as examples of price controls; certificate-of-need programs, utilization review programs, and practice guidelines as examples of volume controls; and global budgets and Medicare's Volume Performance Standards as examples of expenditure controls (Rice 1996). Each of these strategies has met with limited success, but cost-control mechanisms under a fee-for-service system have not been reliable or consistent.

Many population health management strategies are consistent with the volume and expenditure control approaches to cost containment. Demand and disease management programs provide new opportunities to control volume by reviewing demand for utilization prospectively, as with demand management, and by guiding appropriate utilization through disease management. Overall, an environment with expenditure controls such as global budgets may value a population health management strategy because resources will be more tightly managed within the defined budget available.

Capitation Systems

Controlling expenditures under a capitation system requires that costs per person be controlled, the number of persons be monitored, and the shifting of costs between payers be managed (Rice 1996). Two main strategies for capitation-based cost control include the use of HMOs and managed competition. HMOs are paid on the basis of capitation, receiving a fixed payment to provide care for an enrollee for a specific amount of time. Payments are unrelated to how much money is actually spent by the HMO; therefore, if expenditures are lower for a given population of enrollees, the HMO can keep more money from the prepayments (Rice 1996). Population health management strategies are appealing to HMOs because they offer the promise of lowering expenditures for this defined population of enrollees, thereby permitting the HMO to retain more money as a business.

As Rice describes, the managed competition model acknowledges that the market for healthcare services is unlike other markets that support pure competition, and instead allows competition to flourish among players who must conform to certain rules (Rice 1996). These rules include conditions such as providing a minimum benefit package, establishing premium payment limits for employers, and even taxing health plans. The managed competition model might be enacted by the development of health insurance purchasing cooperatives or health alliances that would help establish rules and monitor progress. Although this managed competition model has not been widely tested, proponents argue that costs can be controlled under this approach and highlight success by the California Public Employees Retirement System (CalPERS) purchasing consortium of public employers in California. Opponents, however, argue that managed competition by itself is not likely to contain healthcare costs and suggest that including limits on insurance premiums within a managed competition framework may better increase the chance of success (Rice 1996). Depending on the model developed, incorporation of population health management strategies could be established as part of the rules for interested players with the intent of lowering costs and improving the quality of care for all covered individuals.

Financial Risk

Payment systems for medical care are often described in terms of financial risk. As an example, HMOs accept prepayment for medical services their enrollees may need and are then at risk to cover the costs of that medical care. This notion of financial risk in healthcare is associated with all types of insurance coverage. Insurance coverage provides protection for the insured individual against the downside risk of expensive medical care costs. Financially, insurance is offered for a price, or premium, that is collected, and care is provided up to the limits of policy coverage. Premiums are established based on actuarial estimates of past medical care utilization, which is a very good predictor of future utilization. When predictions about actual utilization are incorrect, the risk-bearing entity either benefits from lower utilization than expected or must cover the actual cost of care for higher utilization levels.

Because many population health management programs have emerged out of the desire to better manage financial risk, health management programs are often linked to risk-bearing entities. Even the level of personal financial risk may be affected when population health management strategies change care-seeking behaviors and the need for medical care. Under such circumstances, the amount of money consumers must pay in copayments, deductibles, and coinsurance rates may be reduced by better health and by better health and care management. Whether fee-for-service or capitation payment systems are in place, there is considerable financial benefit for the entity at risk, as well as for patients, if healthcare expenditures are reduced by better population health management.

Reducing Healthcare Costs

Regardless of type, population health management program development requires an investment of resources and managerial commitment. Justification of this investment is unlikely if financial savings are not expected from a program. Whether a program is developed by a hospital, a health plan, the government, or an employer, one of the primary goals of the program is to better manage health to reduce costs while hopefully improving health and healthcare services. Unfortunately, given the financial structure of most programs, it is unlikely for a program to emerge from the purely altruistic goals of helping improve patient health and well-being in the absence of cost considerations.

Program development is often justified on the basis of multiple goals and multiple potentially beneficial outcomes. However, the high costs of medical care for chronic and catastrophic illnesses are of particular concern for payers. Population health management strategies are attractive to these payers because of a demonstrated commitment to healthcare cost containment that is consistent with their interest in improving health outcomes and the quality of care provided.

Quality

The third major issue in health policy debates is that of quality. With increasing healthcare expenditures, the expectation of concurrent increases in quality has not been realized. As noted by McGlynn and Brook (2001), failures in quality of care result in premature death and needless suffering for patients in all parts of the healthcare system. The Institute of Medicine has presented a definition of quality of care that is accepted by many: "the degree to which health services for individual populations increase the likelihood of desired health outcomes and are consistent with current professional knowledge" (Lohr 1990). Health management strategies benefit by considering this definition as they define populations and desired outcomes for the targeted individuals.

Measuring actual quality in healthcare, however, is fraught with problems. Agreement about which indicators of healthcare quality to measure and deciding how frequently measurements should be undertaken is part of the program development process for many health management initiatives. In addition, defining quality improvement goals for programs and designing a program environment that provides incentives to attain such goals is an important component of program development. Consideration of the different issues in quality assessment and the special problem of medical errors helps to conclude this discussion about why population health management is important.

Quality Assessment

As described by McGlynn and Brook, quality monitoring occurs when one examines different dimensions of the healthcare system and assesses their quality. Performance quality is assessed by either a systems strategy such as total quality management or continuous quality improvement, or by a clinical strategy that focuses on specific health conditions or services (McGlynn and Brook 1996).

Both quality assessment frameworks are important in the context of population health management. Population health management strategies are consistent with a systems approach to quality assessment because they consider the structures, processes, and outcomes of care as they attempt to improve the health and well-being of individuals. Programs are often developed with specific system improvement objectives such as improving care coordination and communication among providers. Also important for many health management programs is consideration of clinical quality. Program objectives such as improving patient health status or improving the care delivered to a particular population of patients are very common. The use of practice guidelines, treatment algorithms, and patient care protocols in many population health management programs is consistent with this quality assessment approach and helps ensure that the care delivered is both appropriate and high-quality.

Another aspect of quality monitoring is the contrast between internal and external quality assessment (McGlynn and Brook 1996). Internal quality assessment involves monitoring quality for an individual institution or program with the intention of assuring and improving its own quality. Population health management programs that define goals and objectives for both clinical and systems improvements can monitor progress and measure success according to those established targets. By comparison, external quality assessment involves comparing quality among several different entities or programs and making the information available for evaluation and decision making (McGlynn and Brook 1996). Benchmarking data, institutional report cards, and accreditation reviews are all examples of external quality assessment processes that affect healthcare organizations. For population health management programs, efforts to compare program outcomes and to evaluate program achievements in comparison to alternative approaches to cost containment or health improvement may be a part of the quality assessment process. It is critical that such programs maintain high internal standards for quality so that programmatic success will be viewed favorably by external observers as well.

Medical Errors

The devastating impact of medical errors highlights the need for improvement in the American healthcare system. The Institute of Medicine's (IOM) report, *To Err is Human*, documents that approximately 44,000 to 98,000 individuals die each year as a result of medical errors (Kohn et al. 1999). Additional studies have shown that as many as 20 to 30 percent of patients in the United States receive care that is contraindicated for their conditions (Starfield 2000; Schuster et al. 1998).

Many adverse effects of medical care itself can also be considered problems of medical quality (Starfield 2000). Errors and adverse effects that occur because of hospital care are reflected in the following estimates:

- 12,000 deaths per year from unnecessary surgery (Leape 1992)
- 7,000 deaths per year due to medication errors in hospitals (Lazarou et al. 1998)
- 106,000 deaths per year due to adverse effects from medications that were not considered errors (Lazarou et al. 1998)

Outpatient care is also associated with multiple adverse effects. One study developed a probability model and estimated that drug-related adverse effects including morbidity and mortality affected between 4 and 18 percent of consecutive patients presenting for outpatient care. These adverse events resulted in 116 million extra visits to physicians, 77 million extra prescriptions, 17 million visits to the emergency department, 8 million hospitalizations, and 3 million admissions for long-term care facilities, at an added cost of $77 billion to the healthcare system (Johnson and Bootman 1995).

Population health management programs have the potential to reduce the number of medical errors and adverse effects associated with use of the healthcare system in a variety of ways. As suggested by Becher and Chassin (2001), part of improving quality and minimizing error must include systems and care processes designed to minimize human error. Strategies that employ care managers to oversee a group of patients can help avoid problems such as unnecessary utilization and medication errors by providing consistent care monitoring, access to care guidelines, and coordination. Most population health management programs are, in fact, designed to address the problem of inappropriate utilization, and thus program success could be credited with reductions in these adverse effects. Additional opportunities to reduce the frequency of medical errors may be realized by having new participants in the care management arena. By having dedicated providers and care managers helping to address issues such as transitions between and among providers and sites of care, the number of errors and problems associated with these situations may be decreased.

Attempting to Cross the Quality Chasm

As described in the Institute of Medicine's report, *Crossing the Quality Chasm* the challenge of the healthcare system in the 21st century is "to improve the American healthcare delivery system as a whole, in all its quality dimensions, for all Americans." Presenting an agenda for redesigning the healthcare system, two of the five topic areas to improve the system are directly related to the potential of population heath management programs (IOM 2001):

- "That healthcare organizations design and implement more effective organizational support processes to make change in the delivery of care possible.
- That purchasers, regulators, health professions, educational institutions, and the Department of Health and Human Services create an environment that fosters and rewards improvement by (1) creating

an infrastructure to support evidence-based practice; (2) facilitating the use of information technology; (3) aligning payment incentives; and (4) preparing the workforce to better serve patients in a world of expanding knowledge and rapid change."

Population health management programs can help to achieve these goals by providing strategies that encourage changes in care delivery as well as promoting an environment focused on improvement. As emphasized by Shortell and Selberg (2002), much of the hope for improving quality in the American healthcare system is to work differently, not merely harder. Population health management strategies benefit from the application of evidence-based knowledge, encourage and rely on the use of information technology, promote the alignment of financial incentives, and help to focus the goals of care provision and healthcare service on improved service and outcomes enhancement.

A further overview of the IOM quality agenda focuses on six factors that the committee notes address key areas for improvement: safe, effective, patient-centered, timely, efficient, and equitable (IOM 2001). Population health management strategies are best designed for success when they also include such considerations, focusing on the goals of improving health and healthcare for defined populations. By attempting to coordinate care and services and focusing on quality overall, population health management strategies can try to do their part in bridging the quality chasm in the U.S. healthcare system.

How Can Population Health Management Occur?

The remainder of this book attempts to answer the question of how population health management strategies can be implemented for defined populations. Part II follows and discusses the importance of defining perspective and populations, and how to target individuals for population health management. Parts III and IV of the text then present specific population health management strategies and discuss how they can help to improve health and wellness within the current U.S. healthcare system. Finally, Part V describes some of the important considerations involved in implementing and managing population health management strategies.

Conclusion

Population health management strategies are desperately needed in the United States. Even given unequal access to health insurance and health management programs, the potential for such programs to better allocate healthcare resources makes them an important component of well-designed healthcare systems. These strategies enable governments and institutions to address the three major components of healthcare policy: access, cost, and quality. By defining a population to be served, access and quality can be measured, monitored, and improved at a given cost level. Furthermore, by managing health for that population, a system can be put into place that helps individuals maintain healthy behaviors and helps institutions to promote appropriate utilization of healthcare services.

REFERENCES

Adler, N. E., T. Boyce, and M. Chesney. 1994. "Socioeconomic Status and Health: the Challenge of the Gradient." *American Psychologist* 49 (1): 15–24.

Anderson, R. M., T. H. Rice, and G. F. Kominski. 1996. *Changing the U.S. Health Care System.* San Francisco: Jossey-Bass Publishers.

Becher, E. C., and M. R. Chassin. 2001. "Improving Quality, Minimizing Error: Making it Happen." *Health Affairs* 20 (3): 68–81.

Centers for Disease Control and Prevention. 2001. *Healthy People 2010.* Washington DC: National Center for Health Statistics. [Online information; retrieved 3/1/01.] http://www.cdc.gov/nchs/about/otheract/hpdata2010/abouthp.htm.

Centers for Medicare and Medicaid Services. 2002. *National Health Expenditures Aggregate 2002.* [Online information; retrieved 3/4/02.] http://www. hcfa.gov/stats/NHE-OAct/tables/t1.htm.

Institute of Medicine, Committee on Quality of Health Care in America. 2001. *Crossing the Quality Chasm: A New Health System for the 21st Century.* Washington, DC: National Academy Press.

Johnson, J. A., and J. L. Bootman. 1995. "Drug-related Morbidity and Mortality: A Cost-of-illness Model." *Archives of Internal Medicine* 155 (18): 1949–56.

Kaplan, G. A., E. Pamuk, J. Lynch, R. Cohen, and J. Balfour. 1996. "Inequality in Income and Mortality in the United States: An Analysis of Mortality and Potential Pathways." *British Medical Journal* 312 (7037): 999–1003.

Kindig, D. A. 1998. "Purchasing Population Health: Aligning Financial Incentives to Improve Health Outcomes." *Health Services Research* 33 (2): 223–42.

Kindig, D. A. 1997. *Purchasing Population Health: Paying for Results.* Ann Arbor: University of Michigan Press.

Kohn, L., J. Corrigan, and M. Donaldson. 1999. *To Err is Human: Building a Safer Health System.* Washington, DC: National Academy Press.

Lazarou, J., B. Pomeranz, and P. Corey. 1998. "Incidence of Adverse Drug Reactions in Hospitalized Patients." *Journal of the American Medical Association* 279:1200–05.

Leape, L. L. 1992. "Unnecessary Surgery." *Annual Review of Public Health* 13: 363–83.

Levit, K., C. Smith, C. Cowan, H. Lazenby, and A. Martin. 2002. "Inflation Spurs Health Spending in 2000." *Health Affairs* 21 (1): 172–81.

Lohr, K. N. 1990. *Medicare: A Strategy for Quality Assurance,* Vol. 1. Washington, DC: National Academy Press.

McGinnis, J. M., and W. H. Foege. 1993. "Actual Causes of Death in the United States." *Journal of the American Medical Association* 270 (18): 2207–12.

McGlynn, E. A., and R. H. Brook. 1996. "Ensuring Quality of Care." In *Changing the U.S. Health Care System* edited by R. M. Anderson, T. H. Rice, and G. F. Kominski. San Francisco: Jossey-Bass Publishers.

McGlynn, E.A., and R. H. Brook. 2001. "Keeping Quality on the Policy Agenda." *Health Affairs* 20 (3): 82–90.

Mills, R. J. *Health Insurance Coverage: 1999. Current Population Report.* Washington, DC: U.S. Census Bureau. September 2000. [Online information; retrieved 8/7/01.] http://www.census.gov/hhes/www/hlthin99.html.

Pappas, G., S. Queens, M. Hadden, and G. Fisher. 1993. "The Increasing Disparity in Mortality Between Socioeconomic Groups in the United States: 1960 and 1964." *The New England Journal of Medicine* 329 (2): 103–09.

Rice, T. H. 1996. "Containing Healthcare Costs." In *Changing the U.S. Health Care System* edited by R. M. Anderson, T. H. Rice, and G. F. Kominski. San Francisco: Jossey-Bass Publishers.

Schuster, M., E. McGlynn, and R. Brook. 1998. "How Good is the Quality of Healthcare in the United States? *Milbank Quarterly* 76: 517–63.

Shortell, S. M., and J. Selberg. 2002. "Working Differently: The IOM's Call to Action." *Healthcare Executive* (15) 1: 6–10.

Starfield, B. 2000. "Is U.S. Health Really the Best in the World?" *Journal of the American Medical Association* 284 (4): 483–85.

Suber, R. M. 2001. "Total Management: Prevention and Management of Chronic Disease." In *Continuum of Long-Term Care,* edited by C. Evashwick. Albany, NY: Delmar Publishing.

U.S. Census Bureau. 2000. *Health Insurance Coverage: 1999. Current Population Survey.* Washington, DC: U.S. Census Bureau.

U.S. Department of Health and Human Services. 1990. *Healthy People 2000: National Health Promotion and Disease Prevention Objectives.* Publication No. (PHS) 91-50213. Washington, DC: DHHS.

World Health Organization. 1948. *World Health Organization Constitution.* (Ratified 1948). *Geneva, Switzerland: World Health Organization.* [Online information; retrieved 8/7/01.] http://www.who.int/about-who/en/definition.html.

World Health Organization. 2000. *World Health Report.* Geneva, Switzerland: World Health Organization. [Online information; retrieved 3/14/01.] http://www.who.int/whr/2000/en/report.htm.

SETTING THE STAGE FOR POPULATION HEALTH MANAGEMENT

DEFINING PERSPECTIVE AND POPULATIONS

To begin the process of population health management, several issues must be addressed. The first is establishing the perspective of the population health management strategy. The notion of perspective helps to frame both the questions and answers of who, where, and why, as addressed in Chapter 2. After determining program perspective, the relevant population for health management must be defined. This chapter discusses these issues of program perspective and population definition in further detail.

Program Perspective

The issue of perspective in population health management is very important. In fact, many different perspectives can be relevant. These multiple perspectives can include those of a participant or patient, an employer, a hospital, a physician provider, a health management company or program vendor, an insurance company, a managed care organization, a community, a state, the country, or even society at large. Table 3.1 shows some of these multiple perspectives and illustrates how defining perspective is related to defining program outcomes of interest, defining a target population, and selecting among different population health management strategies.

From targeting individuals to developing interventions to specifying desired program outcomes, perspective will affect most programmatic decisions. Considering targeting participants, from the perspective of a physician, it is very important to target those individual patients for interventions who are in greatest need of clinical attention. However, from the perspective of an insurance company or other payer, targeting individuals who utilize the most medical care services—regardless of clinical needs— may be paramount. Program intervention development then follows participant targeting. Following this logic, physician-driven programs would likely concentrate on clinical interventions and payer-driven programs might emphasize appropriate ways to reduce healthcare utilization.

Perspective and Program Goals

Perspective is particularly relevant when addressing the issue of desired program goals and outcomes. Outcome measures and evaluation strategies may

TABLE 3.1
Defining
Perspective
in Population
Health
Management

Perspective	Major Program Outcomes of Interest	Target Population	Population Health Management Strategies
Employer	• Cost • Reducing disability • Productivity	Employees	• Lifestyle management • Demand management • Disability management • Catastrophic care management
Society	• Cost • Health • Productivity	Citizens	• Lifestyle management • Demand management • Disease management
Government as insurer	• Cost • Health	Medicare beneficiaries; Medicaid recipients	• Lifestyle management • Demand management • Disease management • Catastrophic care management
Patients	• Health and wellness • Out-of-pocket cost • Improved functional outcomes	Individuals	• Self-care focus of programs • All options may be attractive
Providers	• Improved clinical outcomes • Appropriate care • Efficient use of time	Patients	• Lifestyle management • Demand management • Disease management
Insurers	• Cost • Health	Covered lives	• Demand management • Disease management • Catastrophic care management

SOURCE: McAlearney, A. S. 2002. "Population Health Management in Theory and Practice." In *Advances in Health Care Management* (Volume 3), edited by G. T. Savage, J. Blair, and M. Fottler. New York: JAI Press/Elsevier Science Ltd.

differ in focus depending on the audience interested in the outcomes. While an employer perspective may highlight the importance of returning individuals to work, a societal perspective may be most concerned about appropriate allocation of healthcare resources. Clear specification of the perspective of the population health management program helps to ensure proper alignment of program goals with program activities.

From a patient or member perspective, clinical and functional outcomes may be of paramount importance. Improvements may be dramatic in functional health status or in ability to perform specific activities of daily living as a result of participation in a population health management program. Patients with congestive heart failure (CHF), for example, may find they have more energy by complying with self-care guidelines. Similarly, patients with asthma may find their activities less restricted as a result of their program participation.

Another patient-focused outcome of interest may be general patient satisfaction. When patients are able to change health plans or providers almost at will, providing them with a service such as a health management program to increase their well-being may help encourage plan or provider loyalty among those patients.

From a clinical or provider perspective, improvements in clinical or biologic measures such as reductions in hemoglobin A1c levels or better control of blood pressure may be achievable goals. Such clinical metrics are clearly associated with better health for patients, but patients may be more concerned with functional and emotional well-being than with changes in specific clinical measures. Other outcomes of concern for providers may be physician satisfaction with a health management program or with the healthcare organization itself. Increased physician satisfaction can be especially beneficial in markets where physician retention is an issue.

The health plan or payer perspective may be concerned with broad financial goals in addition to the issues of provider and patient satisfaction. Plans at risk for the medical care costs of their members will be especially interested in reduced utilization and improvements in financial indices such as reduced bed days, fewer hospitalizations, fewer emergency department visits, and lower overall healthcare costs. Per member per month costs are typically tracked; therefore, trying to reduce those costs for the defined population will certainly be beneficial. Even in situations where plans have delegated financial risk to their physician providers, they may be interested in improved financial outcomes as a way to increase physician satisfaction with their managed care contracts and services.

Employers trying to reap the benefits of population health management programs may be interested in broad cost savings, but are also focused specifically on health improvements that affect their workforce. Outcomes such as reductions in absenteeism and lost productivity will be of great interest, whether programs are directed towards employees who miss work or towards their dependents whose illnesses result in employees missing work time. Beyond reductions in sick time, overall reductions in costs related to disability will also be a concern. Better management of chronic illnesses whose burden is reflected in disability over time will certainly be of interest.

Another ancillary outcome of note to employers is employee satisfaction. When employers offer well-received population health management programs, resultant employee satisfaction may help employers over time with retention and other human resources concerns.

Perspective and Program Sponsorship

In the context of this book, this notion of perspective is consistent with discussions of program sponsors. By sponsoring, or paying for, a population health management program, that entity becomes the focus of population definition and other related program activities and goals. For example, when a demand management program is offered through an employer, it is the perspective of that employer that is considered crucial in the definition of the population, targeting of individuals, program parameters, and specification of program outcomes. Similarly, if a hospital is sponsoring a disease management initiative, the perspective of that hospital with respect to patient base, program activities, and program goals is very important. When entities share financial responsibility for a population health management program, goals and program parameters must be clearly specified at the initial stages of program design to ensure that achievement of program outcomes will meet sponsors' criteria for program success.

Defining A Population

Once perspective has been defined for a population health management initiative, the program must next define the relevant population for health management. For the United States, the population can be segmented in a number of ways. This chapter describes seven different strategies for defining populations by:

1. age;
2. income;
3. geography;
4. community;
5. employer;
6. insurance coverage; and
7. health status.

In addition to these different approaches to defining a population, an individual can be a member of multiple populations. Program perspective remains critical when one considers both how a population is defined for management and which population grouping is most relevant for each individual participant.

Table 3.2 below summarizes some of this information by presenting the alternative strategies for population segmentation, describing the rationale for this grouping, and providing an example of this stratification.

Factor	Rationale for Segmentation in Population Health Management	Example Groups
Age	Permits development of age-appropriate health behavior and wellness strategies	Federal Medicare program uses age 65 as cutoff point to determine eligibility for elderly
Income	For low-income individuals, increases access to lower-cost clinics and care options; used as justification for sliding fee scales	Among criteria used for Medicaid eligibility; may define low-income groups for health centers and clinics
Geography	Creates natural boundaries for defining populations	Proximity to a hospital for pregnant women; Medicaid programs defined by state
Community	A subset of geographic segmentation, helps organize outreach, funding, and health information network development; provides foundation to develop community-based health indicators and health goals for local populations	Healthy Cities Project of the World Health Organization; Community Health Status Indicators Project with the Health Resources and Service Administration (HRSA) of the U.S. Department of Health and Human Services; Healthwise Healthy Communities Project in Idaho
Employer	Employers providing health insurance and disability coverage can also target employee groups for population health management interventions	Employee population
Insurance Coverage	Insurance carriers are responsible for medical care costs of enrolled populations, thus their incentives are aligned with population health management goals	Enrolled population; health plan members
Health	Targeting groups on the basis of disease or health status permits stratification into groups who will most benefit from specific population health management interventions	Groups defined by disease status or other health criterion

TABLE 3.2
Defining Populations in Population Health Management

SOURCE: McAlearney, A. S. 2002. "Population Health Management in Theory and Practice." In *Advances in Health Care Management* (Volume 3), edited by G. T. Savage, J. Blair, and M. Fottler. New York: JAI Press/Elsevier Science Ltd.

Age-Based Stratification

One of the more common ways the U.S. population is segmented is by age. By separating the 65+ population from the under-65 population, and then further segmenting the under-18 population, three major groups are defined for population health management: elderly, adults, and children. Age-based stratification is used by the federal government to define insured populations, with the 65+ age group eligible for Medicare coverage. In addition, disabled individuals are eligible for Medicare coverage regardless of age.

Defining populations by age is a common strategy for commercial insurance plans and managed care organizations as well. For managed care organizations developing different risk-based insurance products, the 65+ age group becomes the target population for Medicare risk product development. Similarly, age strata may be used to target marketing campaigns for populations appropriate for different insurance products. Stratifying a population by age gives researchers and actuaries a basis upon which to try to predict healthcare utilization and medical care costs over time. Because the 65+ group is associated with higher utilization than the under-65 group, this population can be segmented to try to measure and predict healthcare expenditures and develop appropriate capitation rates.

Age-based stratification is also important for organizations involved in outreach and program development. The 65+ age group is a common target for adult immunization program outreach due to disease susceptibility and the likelihood of bad outcomes associated with influenza and pneumonia. Immunization programs offering flu shots (recommended annually) or pneumovax injections (needed once every ten years) are established in locations frequented by seniors such as pharmacies and senior centers. Similarly, lifestyle management programs may be varied based on the age group of interest and needs of the population targeted. Fitness programs focused on seniors may emphasize stretching and flexibility while programs for a younger population may include higher-impact activities and more aerobic exercise.

Other age groups may be targeted for different health management programs. Considering younger ages, the pediatric population age two and under is a key group for strategies to improve childhood immunization rates. Childhood immunization programs may be established in mobile clinics that visit schools. Managed care organizations concerned about improving HEDIS (Health Plan Employer Data and Information Set) scores often target this pediatric population in quality improvement studies and develop outreach strategies to try to improve immunization rates. Similarly, pediatricians institute reminder systems such as postcards and telephone calls to encourage parents to complete their children's immunization schedules. Health departments may offer another set of outreach strategies including immunization clinics designed to make sure all residents are fully immunized by age two. (See 3.1 "Population Segmentation by Age" at www.ache.org/pubs/mcalearney/start.cfm.)

Income Criteria

Another form of stratification occasionally used is that based on income. For low-income individuals without insurance, healthcare organizations often develop sliding scale payment options that encourage people to pay what they can afford for medical care services. Healthcare centers such as neighborhood health centers, county health centers, Federally Qualified Health Centers (FQHCs), and free clinics (not mutually exclusive) are organized to provide access to care for needy individuals. These centers accept patients who cannot afford to pay as well as those eligible for Medicaid or those who will self pay. These health centers may not offer patients freedom of choice about which provider they see, but they do provide access to care for low-income persons in their areas.

While not based solely on income criteria, the federal- and state-sponsored Medicaid program is a specific example of an insurance program that does consider income in defining eligibility. Medicaid is not automatically available for all poor persons; however, federal poverty levels are used to define eligibility for certain groups of persons including the medically needy and those receiving some form of cash assistance, such as Aid to Families with Dependent Children (AFDC) or Temporary Assistance for Needy Families (TANF), the AFDC replacement program. In addition, states may define their own income criteria for eligibility for healthcare services or insurance coverage.

Geography

Defining a population by geographic region is another very common strategy for population health management programs. For healthcare organizations, specifying a target market area is an important way to reach potential customers. Hospitals trying to attract new patients have found some individual service lines are especially inclined to bring new patients into the hospital. Two of these lines are particularly susceptible to definition by geographic area: emergency departments and obstetrics services (Roghmann and Zastowny 1979).

Emergency department use in hospitals usually reflects the characteristics of the population geographically near the institution. For hospitals located in an urban area with a high concentration of low-income residents, poor reimbursement for emergency services may be a problem because the population in close geographic proximity is likely to be uninsured or underinsured and unable to afford costly emergency care. In contrast, hospitals located in middle class suburbs benefit from being able to serve a higher proportion of insured patients who use their emergency departments, since services are more likely to be reimbursed.

Maternity care service provision is also associated with geographic proximity to a hospital. With the exception of rural areas where pregnant women may be forced to travel longer distances to obtain hospital care, women are not likely to travel far from their homes to deliver their babies (Roghmann and Zastowny 1979). Defining a market area for maternity services typically uses distance as a factor in planning outreach efforts and marketing communications to focus on a limited geographic area. Billboards, bus stop benches, and radio and television spots are all appropriate communications media to support concentrated geographic market outreach.

Another area where geography becomes very important in segmenting populations for health management is that of rural health management. The distinction between urban and rural populations is important for a number of health reasons including access to medical providers, health status, and socioeconomic status. Residents living in rural communities—approximately one-fourth of all Americans—fare worse than their urban counterparts on all indicators of access to care, health status, income, level of education, and employment. Problems noted in studies of access issues in rural health (Dansky et al. 1998; Kassab et al. 1996; Hartley et al. 1994; Strickland and Strickland 1996) include:

- economic barriers;
- racial issues;
- personnel shortages;
- issues surrounding mental health needs;
- prevention services;
- rural hospital closures;
- travel distances;
- problems related to being elderly and living in a rural community;
- harsh weather; and
- limited access to related healthcare services such as home health, skilled nursing, physical therapy, and rehabilitation.

Population health management programs established in rural areas can assess population needs specific to the area and develop appropriate program components based on such findings.

The issue of geography also affects health insurance coverage. For programs such as Medicaid, state of residence makes a difference and dictates program eligibility requirements and benefit levels. Similarly, state regulations often constrain insurance product offerings, and regulatory climate can influence malpractice coverage rates for providers. (See 3.2 "Segmentation by Geography: Health Reform Initiatives" and 3.3 "Segmentation by Geography: Regular Source of Care and a Medical Home" at www.ache.org/pubs/mcalearney/start.cfm.)

Communities

Moving from the broad concept of geography to the specific notion of a community creates another important set of criteria by which to define a population. Public health programs have been developed around the notion of defined communities for outreach, funding, and health information network development. Specifically, the definition of community provides the foundation for developing community-based health outcome indicators. For health goals such as those outlined in *Healthy People 2000* or *Healthy People 2010,* many individual communities have tried to redefine health goals in metrics appropriate for their own population. Using adjustment factors such as age, communities are able to establish target rates for health improvement that are reasonable and appropriate. Prime examples of such community-based health initiatives include The Healthy Cities Project of the World Health Organization (WHO) and the Community Health Status Indicators Project.

Healthy Cities projects or Healthy Communities initiatives are organized as community-wide efforts to bring the public, private, and nonprofit sectors together to improve community health. Ideally, projects move beyond health promotion activities to establish processes to confront multiple community health problems over an extended period of time. The term Healthy Cities emerged in 1985 as the title of a speech given at a meeting in Canada. This concept was described to reflect the fact that health is the result of more than medical care, noting that people are healthy when they live in healthy cities—environments that are nurturing—and when they are involved in the life of their community. The World Health Organization adopted this concept and opened a Healthy Cities Project office in Europe to encourage cities to target and solve their own local problems, including children's issues, environmental problems, homelessness, safety, education, and other general health issues. The object of the program is to promote collaboration amongst citizens and representatives of business, government, and other sectors of the community. Currently, the Healthy Cities (www.healthycities.org/facts/overview.htm) movement includes projects in more than 1000 cities around the world with new initiatives starting at any time (Kenzer 2000; Lasker 1997; Hancock 1993).

As another example of a community-based population health management strategy, the Community Health Status Indicators Project (CHSI) has been developed as a collaborative activity of the National Association of County and City Health Officials, the Association of State and Territorial Health Officials, and the Public Health Foundation. It is funded by the Health Resources and Service Administration (HRSA) of the U.S. Department of Health and Human Services. This project was designed to provide health and health-related data and present it in a way to make it accessible and useful to individual communities. Building upon community health profiles developed by various state and local health departments, federal agencies, and national organizations, additional data elements enable comparisons and enhance the community health profiles. Information included in these enhanced community reports consists of demographic and health characteristics of individual communities and peer communities; estimates of behavioral risks; preventive service use, access, and health resource use; estimates of the size of at-risk target populations; and prevalence rates for diseases and conditions. Overall, health assessment information has been made available for all U.S. counties, and the information is synthesized to improve the ability of individual communities to develop appropriate health programs and outreach activities to match the needs of their defined populations. (See 3.4 "Segmentation by Communities: Healthwise Healthy Communities Project"; 3.5 "Defining Community in Health Services Research"; and 3.6 "Segmentation by Community for Health Reform Experimentation" at www.ache.org/ pubs/mcalearney/ start.cfm.)

Employers

As another way to define a population group, an employer's employees form a very distinct population. This segment is important because it is this group for whom the employer is typically responsible for providing benefits such as health insurance, behavioral health services, and disability coverage. While the size of an employee population is clearly important, the employee characteristics are also influential and may affect issues such as insurance coverage eligibility or benefit limits. Specifically, characteristics of the population employed will determine the level of insurance premiums that must be paid, and may proscribe insurance plan coverage options.

Employers are understandably concerned about rapidly increasing health insurance premiums and the effect premium increases have on their profitability. Coverage of health benefits, considered standard in the United States, is not consistent around the world. Companies who do compete in a global market note that U.S. production prices are higher because of the level of benefits they must offer their employees. Employees are being asked to pay an increasing percentage of their health insurance premiums, and many employers are considering new health plan options that involve increased employee cost sharing. Examples include plans with high deductibles, healthcare spending accounts, defined contribution plans, and after-tax savings accounts (Martinez 2002). Nonetheless, employer-sponsored health insurance coverage remains the norm for most large and mid-sized U.S. employers, who typically cover a substantially larger proportion of healthcare expenses than their employees. (See 3.7 "Employer-based Cost Containment Strategies" at www.ache.org/pubs/mcalearney/ start.cfm.)

From an employee perspective, the availability of benefits may be very important in the decision to work for a particular employer. Later, after the employment decision is made, levels of coverage and past medical care experience become important when an employee must decide among insurance plan options and coverage limits. Younger women considering getting pregnant will be concerned about coverage for maternity services such as prenatal care and hospitalization, while individuals with preexisting health conditions such as diabetes or heart disease might be specifically concerned about coverage, deductibles, and copayments for office visits and unexpected hospitalizations. Benefits coverage limits may also be of concern when determining the employee's responsibility for premium cost sharing.

The level of employee compensation provided in the form of benefits certainly affects employee take-home pay. Depending on compensation level, employees may be taking home a considerable proportion of their compensation in the form of tax-free benefits. Whether mandated benefits or taxes, employee take-home compensation is affected by the cost of these benefits (Wilson 1996).

Another employer issue concerning mental and behavioral health is the additional effect these problems have on disability. According to the recent study, "The Global Burden of Disease" funded by the World Bank, the World Health Organization, and private foundations, depression was the number one cause of disability in the world in 1990, affecting 50.8 million persons worldwide, or 13.2 percent of the global population. Three additional mental disorders (bipolar disorder, schizophrenia, and obsessive-compulsive disorder) were listed in the top 10, and alcohol use, another behavioral health issue, was ranked fifth, affecting 15.8 million persons or 4.1 percent of the world's population (Murray and Lopez 1996; Norquist and Hyman 1999). For employers trying to maximize productivity and profits, the problems of poor health and disability within their working population cannot be ignored. Disability management as a population health management strategy is discussed further in Chapter 9. (See 3.8 "Segmentation by Employer: Mental and Behavioral Health Issues" at www.ache.org/pubs/mcalearney/start.cfm.)

Occupational health and safety is another area of employee health and wellness where a focus on the employee population is central. The Occupational Safety and Health Administration (OSHA) of the U.S. Department of Labor focuses on workplace safety and health, striving to make America's workplaces the safest in the world. Established by the Occupational Safety and Health Act of 1970, the mission of OSHA is to save lives, prevent injuries, and protect the health of workers in America. More than 100 million working men and women and 6.5 million employers are covered by the Act of 1970. OSHA reports that 6,000 Americans die from workplace injuries annually and another 50,000 workers are estimated to die due to illnesses caused by workplace exposures. In addition, 6 million people are estimated to suffer annually from nonfatal workplace injuries. OSHA estimates that injuries alone cost U.S. businesses over $110 billion each year. OSHA works to establish protective standards, enforce the established standards, and provide outreach for employers and employees with technical outreach and consultation programs. The OSHA staff includes inspectors, investigators, engineers, physicians, educators, standards writers, and other technical and support personnel who focus on reducing workplace injuries and illnesses.

The employee population is an obvious target for employer-sponsored lifestyle management initiatives (discussed in Chapter 5). Many large employers sponsor wellness initiatives such as smoking cessation programs or weight management classes for their employees as a means of potentially lowering their health and disability costs. Such health and wellness programs may be developed in-house, or offered through the sponsorship of other interested groups such as insurance plans and managed care organizations trying to improve the health status of their defined population of employees. Available programs range from classes on health promotion topics to health and safety classes such as CPR to healthy lifestyle classes. Depending on the employer, initiatives may also have a clinical component such as health screenings or immunization clinics designed to promote employee health and avoid illness. In general, programs are designed to help both employees and employers by attempting to lower health risks and their associated medical care and disability costs. (See 3.9 "Employer Cost Containment Strategies: Purchasing Coalitions" at www.ache.org/pubs/mcalearney/start.cfm.)

Focusing on the characteristics and needs of an employee population creates many opportunities for health management. This population definition reflects associated segmentation criteria such as insurance coverage, age, and even health risk level, thus taking advantage of the segmentation of employee groups for health management can be very useful in targeting population health management strategies.

Insurance-Based Criteria

Populations are also segmented based on insurance status. Managed care organizations (MCOs) define their enrollee populations as "members," commercial insurance companies refer to their "subscribers," the federal Medicare program defines its "beneficiaries," and persons covered by Medicaid insurance are often referred to as "recipients." Defining populations by insurance coverage enables the insurance provider to specify benefits and coverage limits for the "covered lives" of its population of interest. It also allows insurance providers to target their populations for various outreach initiatives that might improve the health and well-being of that group.

Financially, managed care organizations (MCOs) work with the notion of prepaid services or a capitation rate paid for their covered members. For an MCO, employers typically pay the health plan a fixed fee, per member, per month, that is estimated sufficient to cover their medical costs plus an administrative markup (and any profit that the MCO has built into the equation). For some managed care organizations, risk is delegated to the actual providers who are caring for the enrollees, but MCOs still have responsibility to monitor medical care expenditures for their enrolled population.

The population of interest to a health maintenance organization (HMO) is typically enrollees who have signed up to receive services from a fixed panel of physician and nonphysician providers. Most commonly, individual enrollees are required to specify a primary care physician (PCP) who will serve as their plan gatekeeper, overseeing their use of medical care services and providing a check on appropriateness of referrals and overall utilization. Some HMOs have eliminated the gatekeeper requirement and encourage enrollees to request services directly from providers, whether providers are specialists or primary care physicians, noting that this increased freedom of choice improves member satisfaction without unduly increasing costs. (See 3.10 "Insurance-based Criteria and PPOs" at www.ache.org/pubs/mcalearney/start.cfm.)

An enrollee population is an excellent target for health improvement initiatives because the managed care organization is usually at risk for the medical care costs of that group. In many health plans, members will receive some type of health assessment survey upon their enrollment. This assessment tool is used to evaluate individual members and usually includes questions to assess medical care utilization, health status, and health behaviors. Responses to such surveys can be aggregated by the health plan to help the plan understand their members' behaviors and utilization patterns. Health improvement programs can be designed with this health assessment information in mind. As an example, health education programs may be developed to address members' needs in specific areas of health promotion and preventive medicine (Chapter 5). Alternatively, a demand management program may become interesting for a plan that finds its members often use healthcare services in inappropriate care settings (Chapter 6). Furthermore, with information about specific members, initiatives such as disease management programs can be targeted to individuals who are in the appropriate population groups at risk (Chapter 7).

In general, the MCO is responsible for providing appropriate and effective care for its enrollees. Managed care organizations are under increasing scrutiny from the federal government and health services researchers to monitor and improve the quality of care for their plan enrollees. The National Committee for Quality Assurance (NCQA) is an independent, nonprofit organization dedicated to evaluating and reporting on the quality of MCOs in the United States. NCQA began accrediting managed care organizations in 1991 in response to marketplace demands for standardized quality of care information. A governing board of directors helps guide the NCQA, and its members include employers, labor representatives, consumers, health plans, quality experts, health policy makers, and individuals who represent organized medicine. By providing information about the quality of healthcare, NCQA hopes to encourage health plans to compete on the basis of quality and value provided rather than only price and provider network composition. (See 3.11 "Health Plan Performance and NCQA" at www.ache.org/pubs/mcalearney/start.cfm.)

Health-Related Criteria

Segmenting populations on the basis of disease status or other health-related criteria is also a common way to target persons for health management. Three common sets of health-related criteria used in population health management include:

1. targeting by cost or utilization patterns;
2. targeting by specific disease; and
3. targeting by site of care.

Targeting individuals based on their cost or medical care utilization patterns is often done by insurance companies or healthcare organizations to better manage their healthcare expenses. By identifying patients with high cost or high utilization, these individuals can be targeted for intensive follow-up programs such as catastrophic care management (Chapter 8).

Using specific diseases to target individuals for health management is the strategy most commonly used for disease management programs (Chapter 7). Similarly, carve-out programs often use disease or condition criteria to define their population for management. Catastrophic care management programs (Chapter 8) represent another opportunity for this targeting strategy when the need for care is defined by catastrophic disease (e.g., cancer, major organ failure).

Finally, site of care is used as another means of segmenting the population. The distinction between inpatient and outpatient services is an obvious example of this segmentation process. Additional segments defined by location include options such as post-acute care services, rehabilitation, or long-term care.

Combining health-related criteria in a more holistic approach can also be very effective. From an institutional perspective, an integrated care management or care coordination strategy (Chapter 10) attempts to coordinate medical care services for individuals negotiating various aspects of the healthcare system. An individual or personal perspective can also be important for consumers. Various lifestyle management strategies (Chapter 5) draw upon this comprehensive approach to health management in an attempt to get individuals to take responsibility for their own health and well-being regardless of the population groups to which they belong.

Using Multiple Criteria

Because of the numerous approaches to defining populations, individuals can be members of multiple groups at the same time. As described in Chapter 2, a 50-year-old woman employed by a bank who has health insurance is a member of many population subgroups. She is a women in her age group; an employee; an individual with a certain income level; a resident in a geographic area; a citizen of a community; a member of a particular health insurance plan; and, presumably, an individual with certain health characteristics that would permit classification by health status. When offered multiple opportunities to manage health, the individual consumer must make appropriate choices regarding health behaviors and health risks. Ideally, such individuals will choose activities to benefit personal health and well-being, regardless of the group that is financially at risk for their medical care services.

Beyond membership in several population groups, the application of multiple criteria can also be used to define a population for health management. The U.S. Medicaid program is a complicated and interesting example of how a program uses multiple criteria to define a population. Eligibility criteria for Medicaid are very specific and vary from state to state. For pregnant women and children, there are actually many ways to receive Medicaid coverage based on different eligibility criteria (Schneider et al. 1998). Important eligibility criteria include:

- *Welfare-related eligibility* that allows Medicaid coverage because recipients are also receiving Aid to Families with Dependent Children (AFDC) or Temporary Assistance for Needy Families (TANF), the replacement program for AFDC created under welfare reform in 1996;
- *Medically needy eligibility* defining categorical eligibility based on being medically needy even when assets are just above limits for AFDC;
- *Omnibus Budget Reconciliation Act (OBRA) poverty-related eligibility* that requires states to provide Medicaid eligibility to pregnant women and children with household incomes up to 133 percent of poverty and to children 6 to 15 years old up to 100 percent of poverty;
- *Section 1902(4)(2) eligibility* that lets states use different methods of counting income or assets for poor pregnant women and children;
- *Section 1115 waiver eligibility* that allows states to expand Medicaid eligibility under waivers for special research and demonstration projects; and
- *CHIP eligibility* that lets states expand insurance coverage for children using Medicaid, a separate program, or both (Ku et al. 1999).

Other individuals and groups may be eligible for Medicaid based on a different set of criteria, resulting in the same desired end: health insurance coverage.

Conclusion

This chapter has discussed the importance of program perspective in the context of population health management. Seven alternative strategies to defining populations for health management have been described, as well as the importance of overlapping criteria and populations. Chapter 4 continues to set the stage for population health management by discussing the process of targeting individuals for population health management. Chapter 5 begins the exploration of specific population health management strategies with a description of Lifestyle Management strategies.

REFERENCES

Dansky, K. H., D. Brannon, D. G. Shea, J. Vasey, and R. Dirani. 1998. "Profiles of Hospital, Physician and Home Health Service Use by Older Persons in Rural Areas." *Gerontologist* 38 (3): 320–30.

Hancock, T. 1993. "The Evolution, Impact and Signifcance of the Healthy Cities/Healthy Communities Movement." *Journal of Public Health Policy* 14 (1): 5–18.

Hartley, D., L. Quam, and N. Lurie. 1994. "Urban and Rural Differences in Health Insurance and Access to Care." *Journal of Rural Health* 10 (2): 98–108.

Kassab, C., A. E. Luloff, T. W. Kelsey, and S. M. Smith. 1996. "The Influence of Insurance Status and Income on Healthcare use Among the Nonmetropolitan Elderly." *Journal of Rural Health* 12 (2): 89–99.

Kenzer, M. 2000. "Healthy Cities: A Guide to the Literature." *Public Health Reports* 115 (2–3): 279–89.

Ku, L., F. Ullman, and R. Almeida. 1999. "What Counts? Determining Medicaid and CHIP Eligibility for Children." Assessing the New Federalism, An Urban Institute Program to Assess Changing Social Policies Discussion Paper 99-105.

Lasker, R., and the Committee on Medicine and Public Health. 1997. *Medicine and Public Health: The Power of Collaboration*. New York: The New York Academy of Medicine.

Martinez, A. 2002. "More Employers Consider New Health Plans Options that Shift Costs to Employees." *Wall Street Journal*. January 8.

McAlearney, A. S. 2002. "Population Health Management in Theory and Practice." In *Advances in Health Care Management* (Volume 3), edited by G. T. Savage, J. Blair, and M. Fottler. New York: JAI Press/Elsevier Science Ltd.

Murray, C. J. L., and A. D. Lopez. 1996. *The Global Burden of Disease*. Cambridge, MA: Harvard University Press.

Norquist, G., and S. E. Hyman. 1999. "Advances in Understanding and Treating Mental Illness: Implications for Policy. *Health Affairs* 18 (5): 32–47.

Roghmann, K. J., and T. R. Zastowny. 1979. "Proximity as a Factor in the Selection of Healthcare Providers: Emergency Room Visits Compared to Obstetric Admissions and Abortions." *Social Science and Medicine* 13D (1): 61–69.

Schneider, A., K. Fennel, and P. Long. 1998. "Medicaid Eligibility for Families and Children." *Kaiser Commission on Medicaid and the Uninsured.* September.

Strickland, J., and D. L. Strickland. 1996. "Barriers to Preventive Health Services for Minority Households in the Rural South." *Journal of Rural Health* 12 (3): 206–17.

Wilson, M. 1996. "Wages, Profits, and Income: Politics Versus Reality." *FYI No. 97.* The Heritage Foundation. [Online information; retrieved 1/18/01.] http://www.heritage.org/library/categories/theory/fyi97.html

WEB SITES

National Committee on Quality Assurance:
http://www.ncqa.org

U.S. Department of Labor/Occupational Safety & Health Administration:
http://www.osha.gov/oshinfo/mission.html

American Academy of Pediatrics:
http://www.aap.org/policy/04992.html

National Association of City and Count Health Officials:
http://www.naccho.org

Community Health Status Indicators Project:
http://www.communityhealth.hrsa.gov

Center for Study Health System Change:
http://www.hschange.com/index.cgi?data=01

TARGETING INDIVIDUALS FOR POPULATION HEALTH MANAGEMENT

After determining program perspectives and defining relevant populations, individual members of populations that will benefit from population health management programs must be both identified and targeted for participation. In other words, even with a population defined for health management, critical next steps become determining who the specific individuals are within the defined population, figuring out what is known about those individuals, and devising ways to encourage identified individuals to participate in a population health management initiative. The process of identifying individuals who will most benefit from program interventions is described as targeting.

Population Identification

Beyond defining the perspective and parameters of a target population for health management, individual members of that population must be identified. Population health management interventions designed to improve the health and well-being of individuals within a defined population depend on a targeted identification process so that the appropriate individuals receive the best interventions for their situations. For a health plan population, this identification process may be relatively simple because population definition is perfectly correlated with population identification. If a population targeted for health management is the entire membership of a health plan, identifying individuals for intervention is the same as identifying members of the health plan. Furthermore, databases may exist that contain detailed clinical and nonclinical information about members that can be screened for potential participation.

When members of a defined population must be identified by something other than plan membership data, identification of individuals for population health management can become more complex. Even targeting specific individuals within a health plan population can involve complicated identification processes and multiple databases. For example, if a health plan is trying to target members for quality improvement interventions such as those mandated by NCQA accreditation guidelines, what parameters are actually used to identify the target population? Can demographics information suffice to identify a group such as women over age 65 who should be receiving mammograms? Or, is it also necessary to include service information such as whether or not these women received mammograms? Considering quality and service, one quality indicator might be the rate of follow-up for abnormal mammograms, and tracking this may require detailed clinical results information. Locating appropriate data and designing techniques by which to identify and target individuals for population health management interventions becomes a critical step in implementing a population health management strategy.

Data Sources for Population Identification

Data and databases are critically important to population health management programs in a number of ways. First, participants in health management programs are typically identified from a review of existing data. Whether the data source is a hospital claim file, an employee database, or a health plan member survey, populations are targeted for management based on the types of information extracted from the data. In the absence of automated databases and analytic capabilities, review of paper records or surveys may provide information about potential participants. However, having different databases available and having them integrated makes the identification process both easier and more likely to be accurate.

Multiple sources of data exist that can be used to identify individuals and groups for population health management programs. Table 4.1 presents a list of potential data sources that might be considered. Determining what data are relevant and necessary in order to target individuals within a population is largely based on program perspective and population definition. For instance, if a population is defined by factors such as age, geography, or income, sources of demographic data that contain this information can be used to identify appropriate individuals. Other sources include plan membership, employer, clinical, administrative, and financial data. These data sources and their importance in identifying individuals within a population are discussed briefly below.

Membership Information

One excellent source of data for population identification is *membership information*. Whether from a health plan or other insurance company, membership information is typically organized to provide basic demographic information about individuals who are members of the defined or "covered" population.

As an example, a health plan membership database contains a great amount of information about its members. A program tailored to middle-aged women can rely on membership database information to screen members by gender and age. Similarly, a health plan interested in providing an outreach program for a particular geographic region of its service area could

Categories	Elements
Administrative	Claim number, managed medical provider organization (MMPO) code, location
Clinical	COT ID (Course of therapy identification), ICD-9-CM (*International Classification of Diseases, 9th Revision, Clinical Modification*), CPT (*Physicians' Current Procedural Terminology*), LOS (length of stay), DRG (diagnosis-related group)
Coverage	Coverage type, plan type, identification
Dates	Service, discharge dates
Medicare	Patient identification
Milliman and Robertson	Diagnosis group, LOS target, percentage of admissions
Financial	AWP (average wholesale price), copay/ coinsurance, deductible
Pharmacy	Day's supply, formulary code, therapeutic class
Patient	Social Security number, age, HEDIS (Healthplan Employer Data and Information Set) cohort type
Provider	Specialty identification number, hospital identification number

TABLE 4.1
Potential Data
Elements

SOURCE: Summers, K. H. 1996. "Measuring and Monitoring Outcomes of Disease Management." *Clinical Therapeutics* 18 (6): 1341–48.

identify its members who were residents of that region and then target them according to the guidelines of the program.

Employer Data

Depending on the type of program focus, *employer databases* can provide a considerable amount of information about employees. Typically, demographic information can be available, in addition to information that may be collected as part of the benefits administration process. Work-related data may be particularly relevant for certain population health management programs. For example, if a program is designed to reduce injuries in the workplace, determining which employees are at greatest risk for which types of injuries will help provide program focus and target appropriate participants. Disability management programs concentrating on reducing employee absence must have access to information about absences whether due to sickness, vacation, personal leave, or disability. As with many types of data, legal and ethical concerns about access to and use of employer data should be considered when considering the logistics of population health management program implementation.

Clinical Information

Another excellent source of data for population health management is *clinical data* that are available for the population. Different healthcare organizations may collect different types of healthcare data, and population health management interventions can be tailored to individuals based on available data. Community health centers may have information about immunization status or well-baby checkups that enable them to target effective programs promoting childhood immunizations and periodic health examinations to those in need of such services. In contrast, hospitals collect data on specific clinical indicators such as blood pressure, cholesterol levels, or diabetes status and these data may feed effectively into disease management programs for a population using that hospital.

Ancillary databases may also provide good sources of information to enable identification of individuals for population health management. *Pharmaceutical information systems* such as pharmacy systems or pharmacy benefits manager (PBM) information systems can provide detailed information about prescription drugs, as well as demographic information. This information may be useful to target specific diseases indicated by the prescribing of a particular medication, or to target a population that might benefit from a health management program designed to improve pharmaceutical compliance. *Laboratory databases* offer information about normal and abnormal ranges for different laboratory values and this information may serve as an entry point into a disease management program. Furthermore, when laboratory information is combined with other data such as from pharmacy information systems, individuals in need of particular laboratory tests can be flagged based on a prescribed drug (e.g., a Coumadin prescription requiring follow-up pro-time laboratory tests).

Administrative and Financial Data

Administrative data provide another excellent opportunity to identify individuals for population health management. One example of using administrative data is to select individual diagnosis codes that might indicate a patient's disease status. For instance, a diabetes disease management program may select patients for participation based on finding diabetes-related diagnosis codes (ICD-9 codes) in their administrative data. Diagnosis related groups (DRGs) provide another source of coded classification information, as do ambulatory care groups (ACGs) for outpatient practice situations.

Utilization Information

Another major category of administrative data useful for population health management is *utilization information*. Measures such as inpatient hospital admissions, inpatient bed days, emergency department visits, or outpatient encounters provide information about populations and specific data to identify individuals. Defining utilization events as triggers for follow-up creates a different strategy for population identification. Events such as hospitalizations may be defined as utilization triggers. Utilization data may provide the basis for program goals and outcome targets that population health management programs strive to attain.

The availability and accessibility of *financial data* provides another way to select patients for population health management. A decision rule for an individual to receive intervention attention may be based on a high-cost threshold. Although creating programs based on financial criteria may reflect an overemphasis on cost concerns for the targeted population, using such decision rules to supplement clinical criteria may be entirely appropriate. Financial data systems may also provide the best source of timely information about a healthcare organization's patient population.

In general, administrative and financial data have provided evidence to support a fundamental hypothesis behind population-based health management—that a relatively small proportion of the population (5 to 20 percent) is responsible for a relatively large proportion of medical care costs (70 to 80 percent). Even more startling is the Centers for Medicare and Medicaid Services (formerly the Health Care Financing Administration) statistic reporting that the sickest 1 percent of the population account for spending of more than 30 percent of healthcare dollars.

Table 4.2 illustrates this approximate pattern for different population groups. For an urban Medicare population, the catastrophic 1 percent of the population and additional 19 percent of the population with chronic conditions is associated with almost 70 percent of total healthcare costs. For a commercial population, this ratio is slightly different, with the sickest 1 percent of the population accounting for one-quarter of total healthcare costs (Maher and Lutz 1997).

One way to identify individuals for interventions has been described in a strategy to improve diabetes care (O'Connor and Pronk 1998). Described as the process of developing a registry of patients who have been diagnosed with diabetes, multiple sources of data can be part of the identification process.

An Example: Targeting Individuals with Diabetes

- Examine diagnostic codes from office visits
  - Diabetes ICD-9 codes include 250.xx
  - Require two codes in a 12–24 month time frame to increase accuracy of identification
- Review pharmacy data for prescriptions:
  - Insulin, sulfonylureas, biguanides, thiazolidenediones, alpha-glucosidase inhibitors, and other diabetes-specific drugs

TABLE 4.2
Population
Segmentation:
Enrollee
and Cost
Distributions

Urban Medicare (Non-Risk) Population

Health Status	Percent of Enrollees	PMPM Cost	Percent of Total Cost
Catastrophic	1%	$4,000	9%
Chronic Condition	19%	$1,500	59%
Relatively Well	80%	$195	32%

Commercial Indemnity/PPO Population

Health Status	Percent of Enrollees	PMPM Cost	Percent of Total Cost
Catastrophic	1%	$4,750	25%
Chronic Condition	7%	$800	30%
Relatively Well	92%	$90	45%

SOURCE: Adapted from Maher, K., and J. Lutz. 1997. "Identifying Opportunities to Improve the Management of Care: A Population-based Diagnostic Methodology." *Journal of Ambulatory Care Management* 20 (2): 18–36.

- Assess laboratory data:
  - Fasting serum glucose for levels over 125 mg/dL on two occasions
  - Glycosylated hemoglobin level exceeding 1 percent of top normal limit
- Physicians and clinicians record individuals they have seen that they recall having diabetes

Using this strategy in a managed care organization, 91 percent of all the individuals who actually had diabetes were identified, and only 6 patients in 100 identified truly did not have diabetes (reported sensitivity 0.91, specificity 0.995, positive predictive value 0.94) (O'Connor and Pronk 1998).

Once patients have been identified with diabetes, the group can be further segmented to target health and care management interventions. In this example, patients were ranked from worst to best with respect to elevated glycosylated hemoglobin (HbA1c) levels. Patients with no reported HbA1c test in the past year were sent a letter signed by their physician along with laboratory paperwork recommending that they get their blood tested and follow this up with a visit to their physician. Those patients with reported HbA1c levels were stratified into three intervention groups for further outreach: level >10 percent, 8 to 10 percent, <8 percent. The group identified with HbA1c levels over 10 percent were targeted for intensive intervention because of their high risk for complications associated with diabetes. Nurse phone calls and attention to pharmacologic treatment were both part of the intervention strategy. Results from this targeted identification and intervention process were both clinically and financially notable. One clinic using this strategy reported a substantial drop in the mean HgA1c level for the population and a reduction in the rate of medical cost increases for the clinic overall (O'Connor and Pronk 1998).

Data Issues

Determining what types of data are available to identify population members and target them for program participation is a crucial step in establishing a population health management program. However, gaining access to appropriate data is not always easy. Information systems containing relevant data may restrict access due to logistical, political, ethical, or legal concerns. Once a program has determined that particular data are needed to identify and target individuals for participation, data issues such as physical access, timeliness, quality, automation, cost, and integration may all be concerns.

- *Physical access* to data may be constrained by different factors such as the location of information systems or access to the individuals able and authorized to provide access to the data. The continuing cost of data access may also be a major issue when programs both attempt to initially identify program both participants and then try to enroll additional individuals on an ongoing basis.

- The *timeliness* and *quality* of data are other factors that can affect the usefulness of data in their role in screening individuals for program eligibility. Both the timeliness and quality of claims data are notoriously suspect as tools for patient identification and these issues must be taken into account in program design. Clinical data may be timely, but access to the data may be slow and costly if access requires chart reviews. Accuracy can also be a problem for most data sources. Determining the importance of timeliness and data quality as factors in population identification must be part of program design.

- *Data standardization* is another important issue affecting data quality. Especially when data are obtained from different facilities, the lack of uniformity in presentation and interpretation can be a problem. For laboratory information, as an example, the definitions of what is normal and abnormal may vary by location. Similarly, definition of what constitutes an outpatient visit (time, intensity, etc.) may be variable across facilities.

- *Data automation* can be very useful in the population identification process. Automation of population selection decision rules in an environment with integrated information systems makes ongoing population identification possible and may help to sustain program enrollment over time. Programs that must rely on manual identification of individuals for participation may suffer from delayed and inaccurate identification of potential participants.

- *Politics* may also create issues for data acquisition and analysis, especially when programs rely upon data from multiple sources. Concerns about sharing data among competitors can present access barriers that need to be addressed. The politics of negotiating ongoing access to data to ensure continuous enrollment across providers or insurers may also be problematic.

- The *privacy, confidentiality, and security* of data are further concerns. While both legal and moral standards affect these issues, they are of concern to patients, providers, and payers. New regulations regarding the use and confidentiality of healthcare information were presented in the Health Insurance Portability and Accountability Act of 1996 (HIPAA) which dictated how healthcare information must be stored, transmitted and managed. This legislation has raised issues about how data can be used for case finding and research in healthcare organizations, especially in the context of developing population health management strategies.

- *Cost* of data acquisition is an issue that permeates decisions about population identification and targeting. When more accurate data are available but cost more to obtain, it is up to program developers to make the cost-quality tradeoff in that decision. Similarly, automated data may be accessible, but more costly to access than manual data sources. Cost considerations about initial data acquisition and ongoing program enrollment must be included in program planning discussions.

- *Integration* of different data sources can be extremely valuable from a population health management perspective. By integrating different information systems, programs can establish participation screening criteria, referral parameters, and red flags across multiple databases to identify patients who would benefit from program participation. Multifaceted criteria such as disease status combined with cost of medical care can be defined to flag individuals for participation.

  With more highly integrated information systems across a healthcare system or community, a population health management program will be able to target individuals for participation based on combinations of characteristics. Combining inpatient and outpatient information provides a more complete picture of how an individual is or is not managing health and disease. Furthermore, the combination of clinical and nonclinical information may be very powerful when trying to develop a program for individuals defined by a set of factors such as social support or cultural differences. By using a combination of administrative, pharmacy, laboratory, and hospital discharge data, it may be possible to identify a greater proportion of individuals who would benefit from a health management program than those who might be identified through claims data alone. Furthermore, when data from multiple systems are integrated, defining decision rules for population identification may make the population selection process substantially less difficult than in cases where data are available only in nonintegrated formats. Program parameters can be more specific when information systems enable targeted identification of individuals within a population for participation.

Selecting Appropriate Data

In practice, the process of targeting individuals for population health management is constrained by multiple factors. Considerations for the administrator planning a program include the following:

- *Program perspective:* Who will be assessing program impact?
- *Program goals:* What outcomes will be measured? How will success be defined?
- *Population:* Who will be in the population? Who will not be in the population?
- *Cost:* How large is the program budget? How must money be allocated for program development, implementation, interventions, and evaluation?
- *Politics:* Who will be involved in program development? Will there be access to desired data?
- *Data privacy, security, and confidentiality:* How will these be assured? Is HIPAA compliance being monitored?
- *Availability of existing data:* What types of data are available and at what cost? What is the process to get around barriers to data access? How will lack of data standardization be resolved? How often can databases be accessed?
- *Access to new data:* Is there sufficient budget for ongoing health assessments, member surveys, or home visits? How often will the population be surveyed?

Answering these questions can help facilitate the identification process for individuals who are to be targeted for population health management programs.

Health Risk Stratification

After defining a population and targeting potential members, various methodological techniques can be used to sort participants and make a health management program more effective. For example, one strategy for high-risk population health management defines individuals who are in Status One—those patients who "are at high statistical risk of deteriorating clinically and incurring high costs within the near term, usually the upcoming year" (Forman and Kelliher 1999). As with other focused population health management strategies, the Status One model relies upon the premise that this group of high-risk patients can be identified and appropriately managed to reduce costs and monitor clinical progress.

When sorting participants, the concept of stratifying individuals based on their level of risk—whether for high costs or high utilization—is often applied in population health management strategies. Depending on the nature of a program, two general approaches are common: (1) selection and stratification based on a utilization event; or (2) stratification based on a threshold. See Table 4.3 for a comparison.

Utilization-Based Selection

When selection of individual participants for programs is made on the basis of utilization, identification of such individuals is usually not difficult. Utilization activities are tracked, so it is up to the population health management program to obtain access to these data. Setting some sort of target based on information contained in clinical or administrative data is one common means of selecting individuals for population health management. Depending on the data available and the extent of data automation, this selection process can proceed on a periodic or ongoing basis, using criteria set for the specific population health management program.

These data can be further analyzed to segment members of the population into different categories for population health management, depending on what additional information has been collected. For instance, utilization data can be used to stratify members of a population into categories such as frequent, occasional, and infrequent users of hospital services. Given the association between hospital utilization and cost, population health management strategies such as disease management programs for frequent users, demand management programs for occasional users, and lifestyle management programs to support infrequent users may all be appropriate. The major challenge for population health management strategies under these circumstances is to encourage identified individuals, especially those at highest risk, to participate in targeted program interventions. Careful monitoring of participant health status, utilization, and activities becomes the responsibility of active care managers trying to ensure good program results.

Utilization Criteria *Examples*	Threshold Criteria *Examples*
Hospitalization	Claims cost in top 10% of population
Readmission	Presence of chronic disease
Emergency department visit	Self-reported number of visits to physician
Number of visits to physician	Self-reported poor health status
Disease classification code associated with hospitalization	Classification in group such as frail elderly, at risk of falls
Repeat hospitalizations within 1 year	Reported use of multiple medications

TABLE 4.3
Approaches
to Risk
Stratification

Threshold-Based Selection

Programs that use a threshold to target individuals for population health management often base their threshold decisions on results of a health assessment or on analysis of clinical and/or financial data. For example, one threshold for participation might be a cost utilization threshold such as classification in the most expensive 10 percent of individuals who have had claims over the past year. A different threshold might be the presence of a chronic disease. Defining these thresholds and searching data sources to obtain accurate information about these individuals becomes part of the population health management process.

Thresholds based on health assessment information are also popular. In many health services organizations, health assessments are a common means of evaluating health and well-being for a population of members or patients. Aggregated results of health assessments may be used to describe a population's health status or health needs, or used to monitor changes and improvements in health and quality of healthcare over time (Brook et al. 1996).

The results of health assessments can also be disaggregated as a means of effectively targeting individual respondents who would benefit from population health management initiatives such as disease management or lifestyle management. Specific targeting on factors such as smoking status may be effective as a marker for both cost and intervention opportunity. For example, one employer-based program used claims data to compare costs of male smokers, ex-smokers, and nonsmokers and found considerable differences in overall health costs of these different risk groups (Lynch et al. 1992). These data could be used to target individuals for smoking cessation intervention programs, but could also be used as a basis for risk stratification for the population as a whole. (See 4.1 "Identification of High-risk Individuals for Intervention: Click4Care and MEDai" at www.ache.org/pubs/mcalearney/start.cfm.)

Individual and Population Health Assessment

The ability to assess the health of individual members of the population is usually an important part of most population health management programs. Health assessments are designed to measure or evaluate some dimension of health for an individual, and can focus on aspects of health such as physical health, functional health status, mental health, or social well-being. While many health assessments focus on measuring definitive outcomes such as morbidity or clinical metrics, an expanding focus of outcomes research is now shifting to assessment of individual functioning, including the ability of persons to perform activities of daily living and personal evaluations of health in general (Stewart and Ware 1993). Data obtained from health assessments are very useful in targeting individuals for population health management programs. Answers to questions about health status, activities of daily living, or health habits can help classify individuals who will benefit from targeted health management.

Health Assessment Tools

A variety of health assessment tools have been developed to measure both general health and disease-specific health metrics. The popular Short Form Health Survey (SF-36 and SF-12) derived from the Medical Outcomes Study is often used as a baseline tool to evaluate general individual health and well-being (Ware et al. 1995; 1996). Figure 4.1 shows the SF-12 as it appears on-line. In contrast, condition-specific tools such as the Arthritis Impact Measurement Scale (AIMS) or the Rose Questionnaire for Angina are designed to evaluate the dimensions of health and well-being specifically associated with arthritis or angina (Applegate et al. 1990; Kane and Kane 1987). (See 4.2 "ITG Asthma Short Form" at www.ache.org/pubs/mcalearney/start.cfm.)

As an example of health assessment tools in practice, the Federal Medicare program now uses a multi-item health survey to evaluate beneficiaries' health and well-being. The Medicare Health Outcomes Survey (formerly Health of Seniors Survey) is self-administered and longitudinal, using the SF-36 and other case-mix adjustment variables. This survey is administered to 1,000 randomly sampled beneficiaries, and re-administered every two years. Data from the survey will be used to focus activities in quality improvement, provide comparative health plan information, and to assess health plan performance. Initial analyses have been made to assess the baseline health of Medicare beneficiaries (Stevic et al. 2000). A 15-item health status survey developed by Health Management Corporation (HMC) is also available to assess beneficiaries current health status and

FIGURE 4.1
Short-Form
12 (SF-12)
Health Survey

I.   SF-12® Health Survey

This survey asks for your views about your health. This information will help you keep track of how you feel and how well you are able to do your usual activities.

Answer every question by selecting the answer as indicated. If you are unsure about how to answer a question, please give the best answer you can.

1.   In general, would you say your health is:

Excellent	Very good	Good	Fair	Poor
○	○	○	○	○

The following questions are about activities you might do during a typical day. Does your health now limit you in these activities? If so, how much?

	Yes, limited a lot	Yes, limited a little	No, not limited at all
2. **Moderate activities,** such as moving a table, pushing a vacuum cleaner, bowling, or playing golf	○	○	○
3. Climbing **several** flights of stairs	○	○	○

During the *past 4 weeks,* have you had any of the following problems with your work or other regular daily activities as a result of your physical health?

	Yes	No
4. **Accomplished less** than you would like	○	○
5. Were limited in the **kind** of work or other activities	○	○

During the *past 4 weeks,* have you had any of the following problems with your work or other regular daily activities *as a result of any emotional problems* (such as feeling depressed or anxious)?

	Yes	No
6. **Accomplished less** than you would like	○	○
7. Didn't do work or other activities as **carefully** as usual	○	○

8.   During the *past 4 weeks,* how much did pain interfere with your normal work (including both work outside the home and housework)?

Not at all	A little bit	Moderately	Quite a bit	Extremely
○	○	○	○	○

FIGURE 4.1
(continued)

These questions are about how you feel and how things have been with you during the past 4 weeks. For each question, please give the one answer that comes closest to the way you have been feeling.

How much of the time during the *past 4 weeks* . . .

	All of the time	Most of the time	A good bit of the time	Some of the time	A little of the time	None of the time
9. Have you felt calm and peaceful?	O	O	O	O	O	O
10. Did you have a lot of energy?	O	O	O	O	O	O
11. Have you felt downhearted and blue?	O	O	O	O	O	O

12. During the *past 4 weeks,* how much of the time has your physical health or emotional problems interfered with your social activities (like visiting friends, relatives, etc.)?

All of the time	Most of the time	Some of the time	A little of the time	None of the time
O	O	O	O	O

SOURCE: QualityMetric Incorporated. 2000. *SF-12® Health Survey* Lincoln, RI: QualityMetric Incorporated. [Online information; retrieved 3/2/02.] http://www.qmetric.com/innohome/insf12.shtml

future risk for hospital admissions. This survey can be administered telephonically and is designed to identify individual Medicare beneficiaries who can benefit from health and care management interventions (HMC 2002).

Risk Screening Tools

One variation of health assessment is risk screening. This strategy attempts to identify those individuals at risk for poor outcomes such as high medical care costs or hospitalization events. Risk screening tools are usually brief (8 to 20 questions) and easy to complete (HMO Workgroup 1997). Ideally, these screening tools try to infer the types of utilization events that might happen to screened members, given the individual characteristics of those members including demographics, disease conditions, and lifestyle factors. When individuals are identified as high-risk, clinical assessment of those individuals is then necessary to evaluate their health needs and risky behaviors (HMO Workgroup 1997; 1996).

Many managed care organizations have adopted a health-risk screening tool called the Probability of Repeat Admissions (Pra) survey. This instrument was developed by health services researchers Boult and Pacala at the University of Minnesota and is an eight-item questionnaire asking about factors such as perceived health, medical care utilization in the past year, caregiver status, and general demographics (HMO Workgroup 1997; Pacala et al. 1997). The information collected with this instrument can then be tabulated and used to calculate an individual's risk score (Pra), defined as "the probability of repeat admission" to a hospital. Separating individuals based on these risk scores enables a healthcare organization to stratify members of a larger population based on their risk status which is defined as their predicted likelihood of future hospital use.

Studies have shown that targeting health and care management programs towards individuals with higher health risks can be particularly effective. In a study of the effectiveness of health-risk screening in health education programs, Fries and McShane reported that including such a component improved program results. Health risk and use of medical services were compared among screened high-risk persons, an employee population, and a senior population. For the interventions, a health education program for high-risk individuals (Healthtrac) was used for the screened individuals and a generic health education program was used for comparison groups. Results from this study showed that targeting health education programs for high-risk persons was associated with a 6:1 return on investment compared to a 4:1 return on investment for a program which did not include a risk screening component. These cost savings were achieved from decreases in hospital stays and decreases in physician visits. Interestingly, health-risk scores improved with both health education programs (Fries and McShane 1998).

Health Risk Appraisals

Health Risk Appraisals (HRAs) are another type of health assessment methodology that can be very useful in population health management. In addition to their use in healthcare organizations, HRAs are also used by employers to select members who could benefit from participation in specific health promotion programs. HRAs are typically longer surveys (25 to 100 questions) than risk screening tools, and their increased level of detail may permit precise identification of individuals for targeted programs such as health promotion and disease prevention. Information collected about health habits and clinical or biologic measures enables categorization of members based on modifiable health risks. For example, answers to specific questions may lead to recommendations for definitive preventive actions such as smoking cessation, weight management, or stress modification (HMO Workgroup 1997; Breslow et al. 1997).

Using Health Services Research Findings

Given the incredible quantity of results published in the health services research literature, these findings provide another potential source of information by which to identify individuals for population health management. A study that reports positive results among a population subset is best replicated amongst individuals with similar characteristics. Defining a program based on study characteristics establishes criteria for population identification as well as for program content. Program participants can then be drawn from a given population based on the established criteria and be monitored according to standards described in the research study. Available information systems enable program developers to identify appropriate participants and permit ongoing monitoring within the defined program.

Conclusion

This chapter has continued the discussion of preparing for population health management by describing the process of targeting individuals. Defining the perspective of a program and the characteristics of a target population help to facilitate population identification by establishing relevant criteria by which to design population interventions. Next, identifying specific people for population health management and sorting those individuals into categories based on risk status or utilization helps set the stage for different population health management program activities. Both identification and stratification benefit from the availability of accurate and timely data and the application of health services research methods to help with these processes.

REFERENCES

Applegate, W. B., J. P. Blass, and T. F. Williams. 1990. "Instruments for the Functional Assessment of Older Patients." *New England Journal of Medicine* 332 (17): 1207–14.

Breslow, L., J. C. Beck, H. Morgenstern, J. E. Fielding, A. A. Moore, M. Carmel, and J. Higa. 1997. "Development of a Health Risk Appraisal for the Elderly (HRA-E)." *American Journal of Health Promotion* 11 (5): 337–43.

Brook, R. H., E. A. McGlynn, and P. D. Cleary. 1996. "Part 2: Measuring Quality of Care." *New England Journal of Medicine* 13 (335): 966–70.

Forman, S., and M. Kelliher. 1999. *Status One: Breakthroughs in High-risk Population Health Management*. San Francisco: Jossey-Bass Publishers.

Fries, J. F., and D. McShane. 1998. "Reducing Need and Demand for Medical Services in High-risk Persons." *Western Journal of Medicine* 169 (4): 201–207.

Health Management Corporation (HMC). 2002. "Population Assessment."
    [Online information; retrieved 3/2/02.] http://www.choosehmc.com/
    Pages/Population.htm.

HMO Workgroup on Care Management. 1997. "Planning Care for High-Risk
    Medicare HMO Members: A Report from the HMO Workgroup on Care
    Management." Washington, DC: American Association of Health Plans
    Foundation.

HMO Workgroup on Care Management. 1996. "Chronic Care Initiatives in
    HMOs: Identifying High-Risk Medicare HMO Members: A Report
    from the HMO Workgroup on Care Management." Washington, DC:
    American Association of Health Plans Foundation.

Kane, R. A., and R. L. Kane. 1987. *Assessing the Elderly: A Practical Guide to
    Measurement.* Lexington, Massachusetts: Lexington Books.

Lynch, W. D., H. S. Teitelbaum, and D. S. Main. 1992. "Comparing Medical Costs
    by Analyzing High-cost Cases." *American Journal of Health Promotion* 6
    (3): 206–13.

Maher, K., and J. Lutz. 1997. " Identifying Opportunities to Improve the
    Management of Care: A Population-based Diagnostic Methodology."
    Journal of Ambulatory Care Management 20 (2):18–36.

O'Connor, P. J., and N. P. Pronk. 1998. "Integrating Population Health Concepts,
    Clinical Guidelines, and Ambulatory Medical Systems to Improve
    Diabetes Care." *Journal of Ambulatory Care Management* 21 (1): 67–73.

Pacala, J. T., C. Boult, R. L. Reed, and E. Aliberti. 1997. "Predictive Validity of
    the Pra Instrument Among Older Recipients of Managed Care." *Journal
    of the American Geriatrics Society* 45 (5): 614–17.

QualityMetric Incorporated. 2000. *SF-12® Health Survey.* Lincoln, RI:
    QualityMetric Incorporated. [Online information; retrieved 3/2/02.]
    http://www.qmetric.com/innohome/insf12.shtml and http://www.
    qmetric.com/innohome/inasthma.shtml.

Stevic, M. O., S. C. Haffer, J. Cooper, R. Adams, and J. Michael. 2000. "How
    Healthy ARE Our Seniors? Baseline Results from the Medicare Health
    Outcomes Survey." *Journal of Clinical Outcomes Management* 7 (8): 39–42.

Stewart, A. L., and J. E. Ware, Jr. 1992. *Measuring Functioning and Well-Being: The
    Medical Outcomes Study Approach.* Durham, NC: Duke University Press.

Summers, K. H. 1996. "Measuring and Monitoring Outcomes of Disease
    Management." *Clinical Therapeutics* 18 (6): 1341–48.

Ware, J. E., M. Kosinski, and S. Keller. 1996. "A 12-Item Short-Form Health
    Survey (SF-12): Construction of Scales and Preliminary Tests of
    Reliability and Validity." *Medical Care* 32 (3): 220–33.

Ware, J. E., M. Kosinski, and S. Keller. 1995. *SF-12: How to Score the SF-12
    Physical and Mental Health Summary Scales.* Boston, MA: The Health
    Institute, New England Medical Center.

STRATEGIES FOR POPULATION HEALTH MANAGEMENT

LIFESTYLE MANAGEMENT

T he importance of focusing on consumers in healthcare is becoming more evident as individuals take more responsibility for their health and medical care. Patients often seek their own healthcare information through conversations with friends and colleagues, the Internet, the media, and other available educational sources. This growing tendency of individuals to become involved in their health decisions bodes well for the success of many population health management strategies.

In the health services sector, an individual or self-care focus in health can be described as *lifestyle management*. This term recognizes the importance of personal choices about health behaviors and lifestyle as they affect individual health. Also important in lifestyle management are the related concepts of health promotion and health risk reduction. Health promotion programs attempt to help individuals make behavioral changes that will improve their health and well-being. Consistent with the goals of lifestyle management, the concept of health promotion includes the notions of attempting to promote health, prevent illness, and protect individuals from harm by changing human behavior and environmental factors (Elder et al. 1994). Lifestyle management strategies utilize health promotion techniques such as behavior modification and education to attain health improvement goals within defined populations.

The concept of health risk reduction recognizes the increasing amount of evidence about the associations between individual choices and health risks and the medical care demand and costs that may result from these risks. These factors also support the impetus to consider lifestyle management strategies. The clear link between smoking and disease as well as other associations between diet, exercise, and health all strengthen the case for lifestyle management programs. An expanding body of scientific evidence has now demonstrated the importance of quitting smoking to avoid risks such as lung cancer, emphysema, and heart disease. Correspondingly, the important role of a smoking cessation or tobacco control program as a population health management strategy is clear. Similarly, reports about poor health habits such as driving in motor vehicles without seatbelts or riding motorcycles or bicycles without helmets provide opportunities for public health education about risk reduction.

Lifestyle management strategies can be appealing to almost any program sponsor. As described in Chapter 3, program perspective helps define program outcomes of interest, and lifestyle management strategies can address multiple goals such as improving health and reducing costs. Employers may be interested in reducing costs and disability while increasing productivity for their employee population. From another perspective, providers may be concerned about improving clinical outcomes and using their time more efficiently. Lifestyle management strategies can be devised to address these varied concerns, and alternative program designs have demonstrated considerable success in improving health and reducing costs.

Focus on Individuals

Lifestyle management strategies focus mainly on healthy individuals who are members of the defined population targeted. These individuals make choices about their behaviors and health risks that affect their need and demand for medical care. Lifestyle management program results are highly dependent on the actions taken by involved individual participants. By capitalizing on the personal responsibility of these individuals for their health decisions, lifestyle management strategies attempt to help such persons make optimal health and behavior choices.

Much of the difficulty of applying a lifestyle management strategy is in getting individuals to participate and commit to the attitude and behavior changes required by such programs. Clearly, quitting smoking or losing weight are not simple choices for most people. Instead, comprehensive programs have been developed to help such individuals make these choices and behavior changes. Many lifestyle management strategies draw from the field of psychology and recognize the importance of individuals' perceptions, motivations, and social circumstances as part of their programmatic approach. Sensitivity to the difficulty of personal behavior change can help programs succeed in the face of challenging health and behavior problems.

Prevention

Prevention strategies are critically important to any population health management program and are central in a lifestyle management approach. Not only can such strategies be used to prevent disease, they can also be used to slow the progression of illness when disease is unavoidable. Preventive services have been categorized into three levels of prevention: primary, secondary, and tertiary (Schmidt 1994). *Primary prevention* activities are those designed to prevent disease or illness from initial occurrence. *Secondary prevention* strategies are devised to detect diseases before the appearance of symptoms, or when the disease is in an early, treatable phase. Finally, *tertiary prevention* activities are used to slow the progression of disease when it is symptomatic and to promote rehabilitation from disease or illness (Schmidt 1994; Suber 2001).

A lifestyle management strategy can incorporate different levels of prevention but will typically focus on primary and secondary prevention strategies. An initiative emphasizing healthy lifestyles may be developed based on primary prevention and target overweight individuals with programs that emphasize weight management and stress reduction. Similarly, specific health education or health promotion programs for adults over age 65 may highlight the importance of annual immunizations against influenza and an immunization every ten years against pneumonia. Secondary prevention strategies are also very valuable in lifestyle management programs. Over 60 potentially preventable conditions and diseases have been identified by the U.S. Preventive Services Task Force (1996) that has established guidelines for clinical screenings. Using a lifestyle management strategy, members of a defined population can be informed about their need for regular health screenings for chronic conditions. These individuals can be encouraged to have annual physical examinations or to attend health clinics where they can be tested for high blood pressure, high cholesterol, and high blood sugar (Suber 2001).

Different levels of prevention may be used in other population health management strategies as well. Demand management programs may include a strong primary prevention component as they target members for appropriately timed immunizations. Disability management programs may similarly include primary prevention strategies as they promote behavior changes such as smoking cessation and weight reduction as part of an overall health improvement program. Secondary prevention strategies such as health screenings may also be promoted as part of a demand management program, or as part of a disability management program emphasizing regular physician visits. Disease management programs specifically incorporate tertiary prevention strategies as they attempt to better manage diseases and avoid complications associated with disease. A diabetes management program will include components such as monitoring blood sugar, annual eye exams to screen for diabetic retinopathy, and regular foot exams to reduce the likelihood of health problems due to diabetic neuropathy. Also using tertiary prevention strategies, catastrophic care management programs and disability management programs will devise targeted strategies to help patients with rehabilitation and to improve long-term quality of life.

Cost-Effectiveness of Prevention Strategies

While many medical care interventions are extremely expensive, prevention strategies are often both inexpensive and effective. Many prevention strategies have demonstrated that they save more money than they cost. Alternatively, other prevention strategies and interventions cost more money than they save, but their cost is associated with incremental beneficial health effects so that they are defined to be cost effective (National Center for Chronic Disease Prevention & Health Promotion, 1999). Establishing program goals for savings and health outcomes given available resources to be allocated can help population health management strategies best serve their target populations.

Cost-saving prevention strategies should be included in a population health management approach that targets individuals and groups at risk for such diseases or injuries. Many of these interventions fit especially well within the definition of lifestyle management programs. Programs promoting screening for nutrition, for example, have shown that every dollar spent on nutrition screening is associated with $3.25 in savings (Nutrition Screening Initiative 1994). A varicella vaccination program for children was estimated to save more than $5 for every dollar invested in the program, with savings driven by both lower medical costs and lower work-loss costs associated with caregiver time lost from work. Considering only the medical costs of the healthcare payer, the program was still shown to be cost-effective. Results showed that costs were approximately $2 per case of chickenpox prevented, or $2,500 per life-year saved (Lieu et al. 1994a). Another study demonstrated the cost-effectiveness of vaccinating elderly persons against pneumococcal bacteremia and found that the program saved $8.27 in medical costs per person vaccinated (Sisk et al. 1997). (See 5.1 "Cost-effective Prevention Strategies" at www.ache.org/pubs/mcalearney/ start.cfm.)

The Centers for Disease Control and Prevention have compiled a report outlining the benefits of 19 strategies designed to prevent disease and injury by promoting healthy lifestyles. Figure 5.1 lists the target areas they report will benefit from prevention strategies. Among these 19 target areas, the achievable health outcomes vary. For bicycle-related head injuries, for example, the goal is prevention of head injuries among children ages 5 to 16. Dental programs attempt to prevent cavities, and smoking cessation programs try to add life-years. Screening programs are designed to save life-years among those screened, and goals are specified for breast cancer, cervical cancer, colorectal cancer, HIV/AIDS, and neural tube defects. Other strategies focus on treatment of identified cases such as sickle cell disease and tuberculosis (CDC 1999). Including these target areas in a population management strategy when appropriate can maximize health outcomes and reduce costs for different defined populations.

A lifestyle management program can include prevention strategies in whatever context is appropriate. Given the population defined and the budgetary resources available, programs can be tailored to the characteristics of that population. By including program elements such as education, health promotion, and screenings, lifestyle management programs can touch every member of a defined population. Messages about the importance of immunizations, healthy lifestyles, and reducing health risks can be sent and received in the context of health awareness and health improvement.

1. Bicycle-related head injuries

2. Breast cancer

3. Cervical cancer

4. Childhood lead poisoning

5. Childhood vaccine-preventable diseases

6. Chlamydia-related infertility

7. Colorectal cancer

8. Coronary heart disease

9. Dental cavities

10. Diabetic retinopathy

11. HIV/AIDS transmission

12. Influenza among elderly persons

13. Low birthweight

14. Neural tube defects

15. Perinatal Hepatitis B

16. Pneumococcal disease

17. Sickle cell disease

18. Smoking

19. Tuberculosis

FIGURE 5.1
Target Areas to Promote Prevention (CDC 1999)

Health Behavior Change Strategies

Lifestyle management strategies can be fundamental components of many approaches to population health management and rely largely on intervention techniques to motivate changes in health behaviors. In practice, four major categories of interventions are used to promote health behavior change (Elder et al. 1994):

1. Education
2. Motivation
3. Training
4. Marketing

Used singly or in combination, these techniques can help individuals and groups make changes in their lifestyles to promote health and well-being. Table 5.1 summarizes this discussion and highlights the differences between the four interventional techniques.

	Health Behavior Change Strategy	Intervention Techniques	Evidence of Effectiveness
TABLE 5.1 Health Behavior Change Strategies	**Education:** to change knowledge, attitudes, and behaviors	• Define educational objectives (cognitive, affective, psychomotor) (Bloom 1956) • Clarify outcomes expected, and criteria to measure effectiveness (Elder et al. 1994) • Develop education programs • Improve understanding of condition • Increase ability to assess and self-manage symptoms	• Self-care information provided to asthmatics reduced hospital stays by 54% and readmission rates by 75% (Mayo et al. 1990) • Hemophiliac education program reduced outpatient visits by 76%, reduced healthcare costs by 45% (Levine and Britten 1973)
	Motivation: behavior modification strategies to alter behaviors, strengthening adaptive behaviors and weakening maladaptive behaviors (Elder et al. 1994)	• Determine appropriate motivational strategies and develop interventions to support motivation • Positive reinforcement • Negative reinforcement • Response facilitation • Punishment • Response costs • Extinction (Elder et al. 1994)	• Positive reinforcement in adolescent weight management program (Coates and Thoreson 1978) • Negative reinforcement in China's One-Child Family Policy
	Training: to develop new behaviors in individuals that will promote health and well-being	• Apply skills training approach including six component steps: • Instruction • Modeling • Practice • Feedback • Reinforcement • Homework (Elder et al. 1994)	• Arthritis self-help course from Stanford University trained participants to care for themselves and reduced visits to physicians by 40% (Lorig et al. 1993) • Use of training techniques to develop skills in health workers such as CPR or First Aid
	Marketing: to build program awareness, increase demand for health promotion programs, and to help change behavior (Elder et al. 1994)	• Component activities of social marketing and health communication • Designed to address large populations of people with a health behavior change message (Elder et al. 1994)	• Social marketing to increase acceptability for a practice or a social idea (Kotter 1982) such as practicing safe sex or stopping smoking • Health communications using mass media interventions to communicate messages about health risks and choices about healthy behaviors

Education

Educational techniques are a fundamental component of most lifestyle management strategies. Traditional approaches to health education involved focusing on changing knowledge and attitudes and were less concerned about changing individual behaviors. However, health promotion and lifestyle management concepts now include all three of these goals with the ultimate objective of improving individual and population health.

In developing educational interventions, specific objectives must be established to provide the parameters for the intervention process. Bloom's classic work describing a taxonomy of educational objectives lists three categories of objectives: cognitive, affective, and psychomotor (Bloom 1956). This classification system has helped clarify the particular outcomes expected for educational interventions as well as provide criteria by which effectiveness can be evaluated (Elder et al. 1994). By specifying educational objectives, lifestyle management interventions can be focused to produce the cognitive, affective, and psychomotor behavior changes desired.

Education programs designed for groups or individuals can be very effective methods of teaching patients about self-management of chronic diseases. While disease management programs focus on the combined clinical and behavioral management of chronic illnesses, lifestyle management programs concentrate on educating patients about self-management of their conditions. Health management programs addressing conditions such as asthma, arthritis, diabetes, hypertension, and heart disease have been developed in a variety of settings. Educational interventions are designed to improve patients' understanding of their conditions as well as their ability to assess and manage their symptoms to help reduce utilization and medical care costs.

One successful program using an educational intervention provided self-care information for asthmatics who were admitted to a hospital. Providing this information helped patients learn better self-management techniques and resulted in a 75 percent reduction in readmission rates and 54 percent shorter lengths of hospital stays compared to previous utilization figures for this population (Mayo et al. 1990). Similarly, an educational program directed at hemophiliacs taught these individuals to self-administer blood byproducts. This intervention resulted in a 76 percent decrease in outpatient visits and a 45 percent reduction in healthcare costs overall (Levine and Britten 1973).

An alternative educational approach to lifestyle management is the patient education center. Whether based in a hospital, clinic, mall, or employer office, patient education centers offer a wide variety of reference materials including brochures, articles, videotapes, and online retrieval services to supplement existing patient knowledge (Montrose 1995). Incorporating this educational information into a well-researched and well-maintained institutional website provides another opportunity to deliver appropriate education material directly to interested patients in need of such information.

Motivation

Motivation, a second approach to health behavior change, is often described as behavior modification. Behaviors consist of activities that are observable and can be defined objectively. As an example, smoking is a behavior that consists of picking up a cigarette, lighting it, putting the cigarette in one's mouth, drawing in smoke, and exhaling smoke (Elder et al. 1994). By using principles from learning theory to change relationships between the environment and certain behaviors, behaviors can be successfully modified. Ideally, adaptive behaviors are strengthened and maladaptive behaviors are weakened Motivation is critical in behavior modification and behaviors can be increased, decreased, or maintained as a result of individual motivation for change (Elder et al. 1994).

The processes involved in motivation include six categories:

1. Positive reinforcement
2. Negative reinforcement
3. Response facilitation
4. Punishment
5. Response cost
6. Extinction

The first three of these categories include procedures that can strengthen or increase adaptive behaviors. In contrast, punishment, response cost, and extinction can weaken or eliminate maladaptive behaviors (Elder et al. 1994). Not surprisingly, the selection of behavioral modification or motivation procedures in lifestyle management programs is dependent on the types of behaviors that need changing.

Each of these motivation processes has shown success in helping to promote individual and population health. As an example of *positive reinforcement,* a weight management program for adolescents gave allowance money to participants on a daily basis when they sustained progressive weight loss (Coates and Thoreson 1978). An example of *negative reinforcement* was used on a nationwide basis in China with the development of their One-Child Family Policy. By establishing various threats about losing job status, preferred residential locations, and work benefits, parents were encouraged to practice birth control and plan families with only one child. A *response cost* technique is used when smoking cessation programs emphasize the negative aspects of smoking such as bad breath, clothing odors, and the loss of personal attractiveness. Developing appropriate strategies for increasing or decreasing motivation is part of program design and depends on both the characteristics of the target population and the behavior change goals established.

Training

Training techniques involve encouraging new behaviors in individuals to promote health and well-being. Applying skills training approaches is especially effective in groups of individuals where people can learn from each other as well as practice the new behaviors they are trying to develop. Skills training strategies include the following six components (Elder et al. 1994).

1. *Instruction* is defined as the traditional form of teaching used in classes. Formal skills may be presented and described verbally, including providing examples of where the skills may be appropriately used.
2. *Modeling* is used to clarify descriptions provided in the instruction phase by demonstrating the skill behaviors.
3. *Practice* in the form of role playing is used to permit participants to experiment with the new skill.
4. *Feedback* about the appropriateness and effectiveness of the behavior is given to the individual practicing the new skill by the trainer and other participants.
5. *Reinforcement* is provided as a type of rewarding feedback and may be verbal, interpersonal, or associated with some sort of material reward.
6. *Homework* is provided to encourage individuals to practice the new skill outside the training session.

Selecting skills training as a way to encourage the development of appropriate health behaviors can be very effective. Training is often used in the development of new skills for health workers. It can be used in a variety of lifestyle management programs such as learning relaxation techniques or can be used to develop concrete skills such as CPR training or First Aid. The arthritis self-help course created by researchers at Stanford University provides an excellent example of a training intervention. Designed to help arthritis sufferers better manage their condition, the course provided a series of classes two hours per week for six weeks. Participants were taught how to take better charge of their care and learned from other participating patients who suffered from the same condition. Results of the program were substantial—participants made 40 percent fewer visits to physicians even four years after the program had ended (Lorig et al. 1993).

Marketing

The fourth technique used to support health behavior change is marketing. Including the concepts of both social marketing and health communication, marketing helps to build program awareness, increase demand for health promotion programs, and helps directly change behavior (Elder et al. 1994). Lifestyle management programs rely on marketing techniques to address large populations of people with specific health behavior change goals.

Social marketing is defined as the "design, implementation, and control of programs seeking to increase the acceptability of a social idea or practice in a target population" (Kotter 1982). Related to the fields of advertising and communications, social marketing attempts to use marketing techniques to change individual and social behavior. Lifestyle management initiatives can use social marketing techniques to promote messages about healthy behaviors and socially valued behavior changes such as when actors are used to encourage parents to spend time with their children or models are used to ask people to stop smoking.

Health communications are another marketing strategy used to promote health behavior change. A health communications plan including components such as a market analysis; market segmentation; marketing strategy; materials and products distribution; a training, monitoring, and evaluation plan; and a management plan, timetable, and budget (Elder et al. 1994) can be effectively used to target individuals with a health behavior change message. In addition to planning, health communications includes steps such as selecting channels; developing products and materials; pretesting materials and making revisions; training; implementing; and monitoring and evaluating the impact of the communications (Elder et al. 1994). Health communications campaigns are increasingly using mass media through channels such as print and broadcast media. Public service announcements, targeted news stories, and even story lines in television dramas have all been used to communicate messages to the public about health risks and healthy behaviors.

Lifestyle Management Program Effectiveness

A variety of factors may impact the effectiveness of lifestyle management programs. First among these is access to such programs. Due to the nature of population health management strategies, the first step in developing these programs is defining a population. Individuals outside that defined population may not have access to health management programs and services, no matter how effective, because they are not part of the population targeted.

Beyond access, however, other factors can also affect the success of lifestyle management programs. Individual characteristics and circumstances will clearly affect whether participants will be willing and ready to make desired health behavior changes. Clearly, access to programs and care does not guarantee that individuals who could benefit from such services will actually receive them. For an immunization program, for example, access alone does not guarantee that children will be immunized. In addition to financial and medical care access, one study showed that additional factors such as parents' knowledge of immunizations being due, having a large number of children, and not having a regular doctor were associated with delayed immunizations in children (Lieu et al. 1994b).

As previously described, the availability of accurate information about potential and included participants can also affect a program by appropriately (or inappropriately) targeting individuals for interventions. Lifestyle management programs have shown marked success when individuals are matched with appropriate interventions based on their willingness and readiness to change health behaviors. The Transtheoretical Model of Health Behavior Change developed by Prochaska and Velicer established six distinct stages of change that are associated with progress in altering health behaviors: precontemplation, contemplation, preparation, action, maintenance, and termination (Prochaska et al. 1992; Prochaska et al. 1994). Distinguishing among individuals who are in the precontemplative stage (40 percent), contemplative stage (40 percent), or preparation stage (20 percent), can help provide a raise for tailoring lifestyle management interventions to participants (Prochaska and Velicer 1997) and help maximize health outcome improvement.

The ability to monitor individual programs and provide feedback to participants in a program is also important. This monitoring process becomes especially important when lifestyle management techniques include a staged behavior change model, as described above. By monitoring individual stages of change and checking progression through these stages, programs can more appropriately tailor feedback and stage interventions to meet the needs of individual participants. Applying this theoretical support in practice enables programs to provide a form of mass customization (Davis 1996) as communications and interventions are modified based on findings about participants' willingness and readiness to change behaviors and lifestyles.

Additional factors shaping program effectiveness include issues such as the quality of the lifestyle management program and the skill of involved educators, trainers, or marketers. These variables are, in turn, influenced by factors such as the amount of resources available to develop, present, and promote a lifestyle management program and the level of organizational support provided for the program.

Finally, even the objectives specified as program goals influence their effectiveness. Programs designed to encourage individuals to lose weight may define success based on achievement of weight loss goals, participation in weight management support groups, number of pounds lost, or ability of participants to maintain optimal weight goals. Depending on the outcomes of interest, a program may be effective in reaching its defined goals whether or not the ideal health improvement effect is attained.

The following section presents three examples of lifestyle management programs and describes their effectiveness for their target populations. These descriptions are included to offer specific examples of program components as well as metrics of program success.

Example Program: Smoking Cessation

Health management programs focused on smoking cessation are clearly a high priority (CDC 1999). The course of 420,000 deaths per year, smoking is the leading cause of preventable death in the United States (CDC 1993). In 1993, approximately 48 million adults were smokers. Medical care costs were estimated to total $50 billion with individual male smokers incurring $9,000 more and female smokers incurring $10,000 more in medical expenses than nonsmokers (CDC 1994; Hodgson 1992). Additional statistics show that approximately 3,000 young persons start smoking every day, and 50 percent of these are estimated to eventually die from an illness related to smoking (CDC 1995).

Health promotion programs designed to reduce tobacco use—including smoking cessation literature, nicotine replacement therapy, and counseling—have proved effective in many settings. Clinician and group counseling are particularly useful strategies to change smoking behavior. Clinical trials have demonstrated a 6 percent higher average cessation rate after one year in individuals who received counseling in combination with other strategies, compared to those who received no counseling (U.S. Preventive Services Task Force 1996). A counseling and advice session by a physician as part of a tobacco control program can help smokers quit and is relatively cost effective. For men this physician intervention costs about $705 to $988 per life-year gained, and for women it costs $1,204 to $2,058 per life-year gained (Cummings et al. 1989). Incorporating smoking cessation lifestyle interventions into an overall population health management strategy clearly has the potential to help both individuals and society as health is improved and medical care costs are reduced, allowing reallocation of societal health resources.

Example Program: Employer-Based Lifestyle Management

Lifestyle management programs are often associated with employer initiatives to improve employee health and well-being. Smoking cessation and weight management programs are among the more common offerings, with many showing definite promise and favorable results. Employer-based lifestyle management programs typically focus on disease prevention and health promotion and may include work-site services such as wellness programs. Specifically, work-site health promotion services may include building employee awareness, health education, behavior change initiatives, and overall organizational initiatives to promote health. Work-site wellness programs typically include stress management, smoking cessation, weight management, back care, workplace safety, nutrition education, health screenings, prenatal care, well baby care, and CPR and First Aid classes (Fronstin 1996). A survey of employers reported that 88 percent of major employers had introduced lifestyle management programs including health promotion, disease prevention, or early intervention to support healthy lifestyles among employees (Fronstin 1996). By promoting health and helping individuals to better care for themselves, these programs are completely consistent with the goals of lifestyle management.

Considerable literature documents the potential and effectiveness of many employer-based lifestyle management programs. Multiple studies have shown cost savings based on reductions in the number of employee sick days and decreases in both outpatient and hospital costs (Fries et al. 1993a). Cost-effectiveness has also been demonstrated, especially for programs designed to reduce cholesterol levels (Wilson et al. 1992) and to reduce cardiovascular risks such as hypertension control, weight loss, and smoking cessation (Erfurt et al. 1991). A review of 28 different studies of employer-based health promotion programs has shown such efforts generally save three times more than the required program investment (Pelletier 1991). Such results are strengthened by the solid research design of many studies using randomized or parallel control groups, or quasi-experimental design (Fries et al. 1993a).

One effective employer-based lifestyle management program is that of the Bank of America. A randomized, controlled study of almost 6,000 Bank of America retirees was designed to test the efficacy of a health promotion program in this population. The program consisted of questionnaires administered every six months about health habits; health risk appraisals that were individualized and time-oriented; materials for self-care management; letters written with a physician's signature indicating any special health-risk problems and recommendations about how to address those problems; and distribution of *Take Care of Yourself* (Vickery and Fries 1994), a health promotion book. Results showed that health risk scores were reduced by almost one-quarter after two years of program participation, and savings were calculated at $200 to $300 per year per individual participant (Leigh et al. 1992; Fries et al. 1993b; Fries et al., 1998). A similar program instituted in the California Public Employees Retirement System (CalPERS) showed that the program resulted in lower medical claims of nearly $8 million, or $300 per participant (Fries et al. 1998; 1994).

Example Program: Injury Prevention

Injury prevention programs provide a third example of lifestyle management strategies. Injuries have been described as the primary cause of productive life lost in the United States in terms of lost person-years, exceeding person-years lost from both cancer and heart disease (Elder et al. 1994; National Academy Press 1985). Whether related to motor vehicles, bicycles, firearms, or falls, injuries take a considerable toll on Americans.

Motor vehicle injuries account for approximately 45 percent of injuries that occur in the United States (McGinnis 1984). In fact, motor vehicle crashes are the leading cause of death and injury to individuals between the ages of 4 and 35, at an annual cost of over $100 million (Graham 1988).

The behavioral factor most commonly associated with motor vehicle crashes is alcohol consumption. Of fatal motor vehicle accidents in the United States, alcohol is estimated to have contributed to 50 to 55 percent of them (Fell 1982). Similarly, alcohol is estimated to have contributed to 18 to 25 percent of all injury-producing motor vehicle crashes (Federal Register 1984). Lifestyle management initiatives designed to decrease the frequency of drinking while driving motor vehicles can have a major effect on reducing fatal and injury-producing accidents.

In addition to programs targeted at reducing drinking and driving, programs encouraging seat belt use also offer an important behavioral intervention. The best protective measure that can be taken to reduce the risk of death or injury in a motor vehicle crash is to use a shoulder and lap seat belt. Research has shown that 55 percent of fatalities and 65 percent of injuries from crashes would have been prevented with proper seat belt use (Federal Register 1984). Developing incentives and strategies to motivate individuals to use seatbelts can have a profound effect on population health.

Another example of an injury prevention program is that promoted by the CDC to reduce bicycle-related head injuries (CDC 1999). In the United States, approximately 45 percent of youths 20 years or younger ride bicycles (an estimated 33 million bicyclists). Unfortunately, nearly 250 of these cyclists have fatal head injuries each year and 140,000 more are treated in emergency departments for bicycle-related head injuries (Sosin et al. 1996). Using bicycle helmets dramatically reduces the likelihood of such injuries by around 85 percent (Thompson et al. 1989). Interventions such as counseling cyclists and parents of cyclists about the importance of wearing helmets is both recommended and demonstrably effective (U.S. Preventive Services Task Force 1996; Sacks et al. 1996). Such programs help reduce the annual economic costs of over $3 billion (in 1991 U.S. dollars) associated with bicycle-related head injuries (U.S. Consumer Product Safety Commission 1994). A 1990 Maryland law that requires bicyclists ages 16 or younger to wear helmets was shown to increase helmet use from 4 percent to 47 percent with a cost-effectiveness ratio of $36,643 per head injury prevented (in 1992 U.S. dollars). Developing a community-wide program to promote helmet use was shown to be similarly cost-effective at a cost of $37,732 per prevented head injury (Hatziandreu et al. 1995).

The Importance of Information

Lifestyle management strategies rely upon accurate information to target individuals for appropriate interventions. Identification of specific members of a population is necessary to tailor interventions for those persons. As described in Chapter 4, a variety of methods can help with the member selection process. For lifestyle management interventions, risk-screening tools are particularly appropriate. Simple mailed surveys can provide information about health habits as well as the presence of chronic conditions. More involved health risk appraisal tools are also helpful and may provide detailed information about individual health risks and behaviors. Other approaches such as telephone interviews, web-based surveys, or even home visits can also be sources of health habit and health risk information that may be used to target individuals for lifestyle management intervention strategies.

Program Overlap

A lifestyle management strategy may actually blend into other population health management strategies because lifestyle management programs can be developed in multiple contexts. Employers may include a lifestyle management component in a disability management program that is designed to help them reduce avoidable illnesses and injuries for their employees. Similarly, lifestyle management programs such as stress reduction, smoking cessation, or weight management may be offered as part of an employee health promotion package that emphasizes wellness and risk reduction, focused on the defined population of employees. Demand management programs may also include lifestyle management strategies as program components for participants who are generally healthy but would benefit from health promotion information and targeted health education. In this context, a demand management company may use outbound telephone calls to encourage program participants to make better food choices or to remind them about scheduled preventive medicine visits.

The purpose of this book is not necessarily to highlight the distinctions between different health management strategies, but instead to emphasize the importance of including different types of strategies in an overall approach to population health management. The approach of most population health management strategies is to direct appropriate interventions towards receptive participants, in whatever way such individuals are targeted for management. Lifestyle management strategies tend to rely more upon individuals and their choices about health behaviors and health risks than do strategies such as disease management that focus more on treatment and care processes. Nonetheless, the goals of improved health and well-being for patients can be the same whether the specified framework is lifestyle management or disease management.

Conclusion

Lifestyle management programs can take many forms and be applied in a variety of contexts. Employers may develop health promotion programs, insurers may sponsor a fall prevention program, or the federal government may legislate a seatbelt use initiative. Regardless of the specific approach used, however, the goal of lifestyle management strategies is the same: to prevent illness or injury by undertaking activities to reduce health risks and promote healthy behaviors. By incorporating lifestyle management strategies into a population health management approach, individual health status and health outcomes can be improved for the benefit of the entire population.

REFERENCES

Bloom, B. 1956. *Taxonomy of Educational Objectives: Handbook I, Cognitive Domain*. New York: David McKay.

Centers for Disease Control and Prevention. 1993. "Cigarette Smoking: Attributable Mortality and Years of Potential Life Lost—United States, 1990." *Morbidity and Mortality Weekly Report* 42 (33): 645–49.

———. 1994. "Medical Care Expenditures Attributable to Cigarette Smoking—United States, 1993." *Morbidity and Mortality Weekly Report* 43 (26): 469–72.

———. 1995. "Trends in Smoking Initiation Among Adolescents and Young Adults—United States 1980–1989." *Morbidity and Mortality Weekly Report* 44 (28): 521–25.

———. 1999. *An Ounce of Prevention. . . . What Are the Returns?* Second Edition, rev. Atlanta, GA: U.S. Department of Health and Human Services, CDC.

Coates, J., and C. Thoreson. 1978. "Treating Obesity in Children and Adolescents: A Review." *American Journal of Public Health* 68 (2): 143–50.

Cummings, S. R., S. M. Rubin, and G. Oster. 1989. "The Cost-effectiveness of Counseling Smokers to Quit." *Journal of the American Medical Association* 261 (1): 75–79.

Davis, S. 1996. *Future Perfect*. Reading, MA: Addison-Wesley Publishing Company, Inc.

Elder, J. P., E. S. Geller, M. F. Hovell, and J. A. Mayer. 1994. *Motivating Health Behavior*. Albany, NY: Delmar Publishers.

Erfurt, J. C. A. Foote, and M. A. Heirich. 1991. "The Cost-effectiveness of Work-site Wellness Programs for Hypertension Control, Weight Loss, and Smoking Cessation." *Journal of Occupational Medicine* 33 (9): 962–70.

Federal Register. 1984. *Federal Motor Vehicle Safety Standards: Occupant Crash Protection, Final Rule 48* (No. 138), July. Washington, DC: U.S. Department of Transportation.

Fell, J. C. 1982. "Alcohol Involvement in Traffic Crashes." *American Association for Automobile Medicine Quarterly Journal* 4: 23–42.

Fries, J., C. E. Koop, J. Sokolov, C. E. Beadle, D. Wright. 1998. "Beyond Health Promotion: Reducing Need and Demand for Medical Care." *Health Affairs* 17 (2): 70–84.

Fries, J. F., H. Harrington, R. Edwards, L. A. Kent, and N. Richardson. 1994. "Randomized Controlled Trial of Cost Reductions from a Health

Education Program: The California Public Employees' Retirement System (PERS) Study." *American Journal of Health Promotion* 8 (3): 216–23.

Fries, J. F., C. E. Koop, C. E. Beadle, P. P. Cooper, M. J. England, R. F. Greaves, J. J. Sokolov, and D. Wright. 1993a. "Reducing Healthcare Costs by Reducing the Need and Demand for Medical Services." *New England Journal of Medicine* 329 (5): 321–25.

Fries, J. F., D. A. Bloch, H. Harrington, N Richardson, and R. Beck. 1993b. "Two-year Results of a Randomized Controlled Trial of a Health Promotion Program in a Retiree Population: The Bank of America Study." *American Journal of Medicine* 94 (5): 455–62.

Fronstin, P. 1996. "Health Promotion and Disease Prevention: a Look at Demand Management Programs." *EBRI Issue Brief* (Sept.) 177: 1–14.

Graham, J. D. 1988. "Injury Control, Traffic Safety, and Evaluation research." *Preventing Automobile Injury*. Dover, MA: Auburn House.

Hatziandreu, E. J., J. J. Sacks, R. Brown, W. R. Taylor, M. L. Rosenberg, and J. D. Graham. 1995. "The Cost Effectiveness of Three Programs to Increase the Use of Bicycle Helmets Among Children." *Public Health Reports* 110 (3): 251–59.

Hodgson, T. A. 1992. "Cigarette Smoking and Lifetime Medical Expenditures." *Milbank Quarterly* 70 (1): 81–125.

Kotter, P. 1982. *Marketing for Nonprofit Organizations*. Englewood Cliffs, NJ: Prentice-Hall.

Leigh, J. P., N. Richardson, R. Beck, C. Kerr, H. Harrington, C. L. Parcell, and J. F. Fries. 1992. "Randomized controlled study of a retiree health promotion program: The Bank of America Study." *Archives of Internal Medicine* 152 (6): 1201–06.

Levine, P. H., and A. F. H. Britten. 1973. "Supervised Patient-Management of Hemophilia: A Study of 45 Patients with Hemophilia A and B." *Annals of Internal Medicine* 78 (2): 195–201.

Lieu, T. A., S. L. Cochi, S. B. Black, E. Halloran, H. R. Shinefield, S. J. Holmes, M. Wharton, and A. E. Washington. 1994a. "Cost-Effectiveness of a Routine Varicella Vaccination Program for U.S. Children." *Journal of the American Medical Association* 271 (5): 375–81.

Lieu, T. A., S. B. Black, P. Ray, M. Chellino, H. R. Shinefield, and N. E. Adler. 1994b. "Risk Factors for Delayed Immunizations Among Children in an HMO." *American Journal of Public Health* 84 (10): 1621–25.

Lorig, K., P. D. Mazonson, and H. R. Holman. 1993. "Evidence Suggesting that Health Education for Self-management in Patients with Chronic Arthritis has Sustained Health Benefits While Reducing Healthcare Costs." *Arthritis and Rheumatism* 36 (4): 439–46.

Mayo, P. H., J. Richman, and H. W. Harris. 1990. "Results of a Program to Reduce Admissions for Adult Asthma." *Annals of Internal Medicine* 112 (11): 864–71.

McGinnis, J. M. 1984. "Occupant Protection as a Priority in National Efforts to Promote Health." *Health Education Quarterly* 11 (2): 127–31.

Montrose, G. 1995. "Demand Management May Help Stem Costs." *Health Management Technology* 16 (2): 18, 21.

National Academy Press. 1985. *Injury in America: A Continuing Public Health Problem*. Washington, DC: National Academy Press.

National Center for Chronic Disease Prevention and Health Promotion. 1999. *About Chronic Disease*. Atlanta, GA: Centers for Disease Control and Prevention.

Nutrition Screening Initiative. 1994. *Incorporating Nutrition Screening and Interventions into Medical Practice: A Monograph for Physicians*. Washington DC: The Nutrition Screening Initiative.

Pelletier, K. 1991. "A Review and Analysis of the Health and Cost-effective Outcome Studies of Comprehensive Health Promotion and Disease Prevention Programs." *American Journal of Health Promotion* 5 (4): 311–15.

Prochaska, J. O., C. C. DiClemente, and J. C. Norcross. 1992. "In Search of How People Change: Applications to Addictive Behaviors. *American Journal of Psychology* 47 (9): 1102–14.

Prochaska, J. O., J. C. Norcross, and C. C. DiClemente. 1994. *Changing for Good*. New York: Morrow.

Prochaska, J. O., and W. F. Velicer. 1997. "The Transtheoretical Model of Health Behavior Change." *American Journal of Health Promotion* 12 (1): 38–48.

Sacks, J. J., M. Kresnow, B. Houston, and J. Russell. 1996. "Bicycle Helmet Use Among American Children." *Injury Prevention* 2 (4): 258–62.

Schmidt, R. M. 1994. "Preventive Healthcare for Older Adults: Societal and Individual Services." *Generations* 18 (1): 33–38.

Sisk, J. E., A. J. Moskowitz, W. Whang, J. D. Lin, D. S. Fedson, A. M. McBean, J. F. Plouffe, M. S. Cetron, and J. C. Butler. 1997. "Cost-effectiveness of Vaccination Against Pneumococcal Bacteremia Among Elderly People." *Journal of the American Medical Association* 278 (16): 1333–39.

Sosin, D. M., J. J. Sacks, and K. W. Webb. 1996. "Pediatric Head Injuries and Deaths from Bicycling in the United States." *Pediatrics* 98 (5): 868–70.

Suber, R. M. 2001. "Total Health Management: Prevention and Management of Chronic Disease." In *The Continuum of Long-Term Care* C. Evashwick, ed. Albany, NY: Delmar Publishers.

Thompson, R. S., F. P. Rivara, and D. C. Thompson. 1989. "A Case-control Study of the Effectiveness of Bicycle Safety Helmets." *New England Journal of Medicine* 320 (21): 1361–67.

U.S. Consumer Product Safety Commission. 1994. "Bicycle Use and Hazard Patterns in the United States." Washington DC: U.S. Consumer Product Safety Commission.

U.S. Preventive Services Task Force. 1996. *Guide to Clinical Preventive Services*, 2nd ed. Baltimore, MD: Williams & Wilkins.

Vickery, D. M., and J. F. Fries. 1994. *Take Care of Yourself: A Consumer's Guide to Medical Care*. Reading, MA: Addison-Wesley Publishing Co.

Wilson, M. G., J. E. Edmunson, and D. M. DeJoy. 1992. "Cost Effectiveness of Work-Site Cholesterol Screening and Intervention Programs." *Journal of Occupational Medicine* 34 (6): 642–49.

DEMAND MANAGEMENT

One of the more common population health management strategies is called demand management or demand improvement (Vickery 1996; MacStravic and Montrose 1998). The term demand management describes a combination of self-care services and triage support to help individuals manage their own medical care and symptoms (MacStravic and Montrose1998). This concept is based on the idea that when individuals are encouraged to take a more active role in their healthcare decisions, their demand for health services can be effectively guided and thereby managed. By providing tools such as decision support systems and behavior support assistance, individuals can be encouraged to use medical care appropriately with respect to where, when, and what type of care is needed. Within a defined population, demand management services are key to managing the relatively well population, as well as helping to provide information to all individuals who would benefit from guidance about appropriate healthcare utilization decisions.

As described by Donald Vickery, M.D., a key figure who helped develop the demand management model in 1992, demand management tools such as health promotion, education, and self-care interventions have existed for many years (Vickery 1996). However, putting these tools together into an integrated demand management model helps provide a framework to address the issues surrounding consumer demand for medical care. According to a 1997 estimate by Merrill Lynch & Co. analyst Stuart Goldberg, the demand management industry was projected to be growing by more than 25 percent per year and could cover up to 100 million people by the year 2001 (Anders 1997). This growth appears to be supported by both the literature and the proliferation of demand management programs and individual businesses. Publication of a journal dedicated to these and disease management activities titled *Healthcare Demand and Disease Management* also provides evidence of the popularity of this strategy.

Demand management tools are defined as "population-based strategies used to control costs and improve utilization of services by assisting health consumers in maintaining their health and seeking appropriate healthcare" (Mohler and Harris 1998). A demand management strategy strives to reduce the perceived need for and utilization of expensive and potentially clinically unnecessary medical care services while trying to improve the health status of a defined population (Montrose 1995). Tactics such as finding therapeutic alternatives to surgery, leveraging self-care interventions, and trying to help patients reduce particular risk factors and adopt healthy lifestyles can be part of the decision and behavioral support offered through demand management programs.

When healthcare organizations are at risk for the cost of care, population health management strategies such as demand management become increasingly appealing. Healthcare organizations and other organizations including insurance companies, providers, and fiscal intermediaries can use these strategies to help contain the cost of providing care. Under a common scenario, when personnel and budgets are dramatically downsized, the ability to ensure that resources are appropriately utilized to address patients' demand for services may help such organizations remain financially viable. Providing patients, employees, or members with access to demand management services may improve their understanding of both the healthcare system and their own medical care needs.

The Context of Demand Management

One of the key tenets of demand management programs is to reduce the level of inappropriate or unnecessary demand for medical care. Such demand is attributable to a number of factors, including suboptimal self-care practices and doctor- and technology-seeking behavior that are unrelated to actual medical care needs. As described by James Fries, the notion of unnecessary demand reflects the idea that services are demanded at the margin, where additional expenditures may not provide measurable health benefits (Fries 1998; Fries et al. 1993). This unnecessary demand is further affected by behavioral constructs including *personal self-efficacy,* which reflects a lack of confidence in one's ability to self-manage health, and *learned helplessness,* demonstrated in a tendency to overvalue the potential contribution of healthcare services to health (Fries 1998; O'Leary 1985; Kaplan and Camacho 1983; Connelly et al. 1991).

Demand management strategies are designed to address the multiple components of individual health that affect consumer demand for healthcare services. The demand management model recognizes that four of these factors have considerable influence on consumer demand (Vickery and Lynch 1995; Vickery 1996):

1. Morbidity
2. Perceived Need
3. Patient preferences
4. Nonhealth motives

Morbidity is clearly important because it reflects the level of disease in a population. However, the level of illness in a population or individual is not perfectly correlated with medical care utilization. Instead, between 86 and 94 percent of the variation in utilization is actually unaccounted for when morbidity is considered alone (Tanner et al. 1983; Berkanovic et al. 1981; Andersen and Newman 1973; Vickery 1996). In addition, much of the morbidity or disease present within a population is preventable. McGinnis and Foege studied underlying causes of death in the United States instead of relying on disease-oriented classifications and found that eight of the nine leading categories of disease causes were actually preventable (McGinnis and Foege 1993). Because a great deal of population morbidity can be prevented, ample opportunities for health management clearly exist.

Another important factor contributing to consumer demand for medical care is *perceived need*. Reflecting the importance of an individual's view of illness and the healthcare services necessary to address that illness, perceived need has been shown to be the most important factor that influences use of medical care services. Perceived need can be influenced by a combination of factors including (Vickery 1996):

1. individual knowledge about the risks and benefits of medical care;
2. perceived efficacy of the proposed treatment;
3. individual ability to assess the medical problem;
4. perceived severity of the medical problem;
5. individual capability to independently manage the problem; and
6. individual confidence in ability to self-manage the problem (perception of self-efficacy).

In the context of additional factors such as cultural norms, education level, gender, the presence of social support systems, and general attitudes of the individual's physicians and other providers, this concept of perceived need can be exceedingly important and complex.

Perceived need notably influences the individual's decision to seek medical care. When symptoms do not interfere with normal activities, individuals are less likely to perceive a need for medical care services. However, when symptoms are obvious or combined with the presence of stressful life events or insufficient social networks, an individual's perception of need for care increases. In fact, individuals who report that they have poor health have been found to seek more healthcare services than others, regardless of whether physicians agree with their judgement of ill health (Connelly et al. 1989, 1991; Vickery 1996).

The concept of *patient preference* acknowledges that patients have a fundamental role in making decisions about their medical care. Working with their physicians, patients are responsible for choosing treatment options based on their understanding of the benefits and risks of such treatments. Patient education research has shown that individuals who are fully informed about treatment benefits and risks are likely to choose treatment options that are less invasive, less risky, and less expensive, even when compared to choices their doctors might make for them (Vickery 1996).

Finally, *nonhealth motives* also influence consumer demand for medical care. Reasons completely unrelated to health such as an individual's ability to qualify for sick leave, disability, or worker's compensation benefits may influence that person's decision to seek medical care. The level of copayments can also influence medical care utilization, regardless of individual health (Newhouse 1994). The effect of these nonhealth motives on demand for medical care has not been entirely quantified, nor have interventions been specifically developed to address these issues (Vickery 1996), but they represent another definite factor that can influence consumer demand for care and services.

Demand management programs that seek to improve individual knowledge about health, illness, and use of the medical care system attempt to manage consumer demand for services. By concentrating on the factors affecting demand and designing interventions to address them, these programs strive to improve appropriateness of medical care utilization and reduce costs without sacrificing health.

Predicting Demand

A number of approaches have been developed to help predict who will utilize medical care services. However, as noted above, merely using the level of illness or morbidity in a population to try to predict utilization is insufficient. Methods that move beyond predictions based on morbidity alone try to combine the health and nonhealth factors that contribute to demand. Some of the sources of data for these predictions include consumers, physicians, health plans, hospitals, employers, and public agencies (MacStravic and Montrose 1998). Specific examples of predicting demand are described further below.

Questionnaire-based health assessments, including tools such as health risk appraisals and health assessment surveys, rely upon comprehensive questionnaires to predict which individuals will use costly medical care services in the time period following the assessment. The University of Michigan Fitness Research Center has developed such an approach based on analysis of self-reported questionnaires, clinical information, program participation data, and cost information. The resultant assessment tool attempts to predict who will be high-cost users in the two- to three-year period after questionnaire administration. Age and gender are also included in a final model that attempts to forecast the demand for medical care.

The assessment tool developed from this University of Michigan research includes questions that assess individual attitudes and beliefs about illness and care-seeking behavior in addition to health information. This questionnaire is a key component of a demand management program and has shown success in predicting short-term morbidity, utilization, and costs. However, because the questionnaire relies on self-reported data, issues such as low response rates, accuracy of form processing, and appropriate analyses (Lynch et al. 1996) must also be accommodated.

Claims-based data assessment is another approach to predicting demand for medical care. Claims data are usually readily available and contain a considerable amount of information about services that have been delivered on either an individual or a family basis. Response rates are not an issue in claims analyses, and claims data are not subject to issues surrounding survey methods such as recall bias or other problems with self-reported data.

Models developed to predict utilization based on claims data can use a number of variables for their forecasts. A model developed by researchers at one demand management company relied on claims data and used 15 variables to identify the 30 percent of the population studied who were responsible for 60 percent of medical care costs over the subsequent year. Actual utilization for this group was found to be 2 to 3 times higher than utilization for the lower-risk group, regardless of illness type. With respect to expenditures, those with serious medical conditions in the higher-risk group had costs 3 to 10 times higher than costs in the lower-risk group (Lynch et al. 1996).

By using questionnaires to obtain self-reported data and supplementing this information with available claims data, the ability to predict medical care utilization within a defined population is increased. Incorporating such analytic capabilities within a demand management program is critical in order to be able to identify which participants can benefit from increased attention through intensified demand management services. Furthermore, when information is obtained about care-seeking attitudes and behaviors, this information can be used to help tailor interventions for individuals who need different levels of attention. By targeting individuals for interventions that are delivered at the appropriate time and level of intensity, such programs can better manage medical care costs and improve patient satisfaction and health consistent with program goals.

History of Demand Management

Demand management has evolved in many ways over the past two decades. Marosits (1997) classified three generations of strategies for demand management. First generation demand management strategies took advantage of managed care models designed to control rising costs by using demand-side utilization controls. These strategies used financial incentives to reduce consumer demand for healthcare resources. Such efforts to control utilization targeted consumers and included strategies such as copayments, deductibles, coinsurance, benefit exclusions, and benefit limitations.

Utilization controls were designed to affect consumers' demand for medical care by imposing rules or including costs that might influence consumers' desires for medical care services. While these early attempts to manage demand or, as many insist, manage costs, had some success, they were also associated with issues such as consumer dissatisfaction and complaints, plan disenrollment, media scandals, lawsuits, and even new legislation that was passed in response to efforts to control utilization (MacStravic 1996).

The second generation of demand management strategies was developed to include clinical strategies along with financial incentives. Often, primary care physician gatekeepers were used to help implement the strategies as designated by the payers (Marosits 1997). New utilization controls such as pre-authorization and second opinion requirements attempted to provide oversight from both clinical and financial perspectives.

The newest generation of demand management strategies is described as a personal health management approach that aligns financial incentives, clinical care protocols, and consumer decision support systems with the goals of balancing patient outcomes and resource use (Marosits 1997). These demand management activities are designed to emphasize informed consumer choice and customization of healthcare services for the individuals at risk.

Describing such strategies as a new approach to managing utilization, MacStravic (1996) lists six demand management options that could be considered part of this new generation of demand management strategies:

1. *Health (risk) management* that attempts to reduce morbidity with efforts to improve wellness and fitness through disease prevention and health promotion
2. *Health plan and provider selection* that try to expand employee choice regarding health benefits and providers
3. *Symptomatic and urgent care controls* that use self-care communications and health education to improve consumer health empowerment and knowledge
4. *Elective treatment choices* that attempt to better inform patients and their families about treatment options through the use of videos, discussions, education, and training
5. *Acute condition management* that uses case management and clinical guidelines to help patients and their providers better manage the treatment process
6. *End-of-life planning* that recognizes the importance of including patients and families in both the planing and management of end-of-life decisions and experiences

Each of these options for demand management and utilization control recognizes the importance of the consumer in health demand choices and tries to help educate consumers to become more informed and empowered healthcare users. This focus on consumers is similar to the lifestyle management strategies described in Chapter 5, but the overall focus on managing demand is central to the demand management strategy. The following section describes specific demand management strategies and explains how they are being used in the health services sector.

Demand Management Strategies

Demand management programs often offer a combination of services designed to modify or improve consumer demand for medical care. These may include 24-hour nurse telephone triage service; advice and referrals; a healthcare information library with wellness topics available through audio tapes and the Internet; registration for wellness classes; appointment scheduling; and even network communication with physician offices for other available services. Demand management programs can also serve as a point of entry for patients who would benefit from additional targeted services such as disease management or chronic care management.

Strategies for demand management attempt to help individuals understand choices they have about options for medical care. While health education and health promotion are often included as demand management strategies, this text has discussed those techniques in the context of lifestyle management. This chapter presents two major strategies for managing and improving demand for a defined population: (1) telephone-based triage and decision support; and (2) communications designed to promote self-care.

Telephone triage and decision support services are typically designed to address issues such as perceived need and patient preferences for care as they affect consumer demand. Supportive counselors can also address non-health issues such as benefits and copayments as counselors work directly with patient callers. Communications strategies try to modify factors including perceived need and patient preferences, but they may also have a strong component designed to modify health behaviors and reduce patient morbidity. Descriptions of these strategies and evidence of their effectiveness follow.

Telephone-Based Triage and Decision Support

Demand management strategies that use telephone-based triage and decision support have widely proliferated in the past decade. Initially developed in a format such as an "Ask-A-Nurse" referral program for physicians and hospitals, telephone services now range from advice counseling to provider referrals. With nurses staffed to answer the telephone, these services are designed to provide both information and support for decisions and behaviors.

Telephone triage services are typically established to help callers determine if their symptoms indicate a need for a physician visit. Triage services may also be linked to utilization management programs or serve as an entry point for more structured disease management programs. In the context of demand management, telephone triage has become a key point-of-entry tool for health plan members and patients accessing various parts of the healthcare system. Health plans have arranged telephone triage systems as a way to manage the demand of new and existing members, while hospitals and clinics have also found success trying to reduce inappropriate healthcare utilization.

With most telephone triage and decision support systems, major components include patient information, patient education, and protocol-guided access to different levels of care. Such programs are usually staffed 24 hours a day by registered nurses. Software packages based on clinical algorithms or decision trees are often used to support nurses and assistants who field calls. These algorithms help guide nurses through decision support and referral options, enabling them to provide appropriate information to the caller regarding conditions or illnesses (Paul 2000). Organizations can install such software packages in-house or purchase telephone triage services from a vendor, health plan, or different provider. These purchase decisions are typically made based on call volume and the healthcare organization's plans to move beyond demand management to offer different population health management strategies (Sabin 1998).

Telephone triage and decision support services are used by employers, health plans, and other risk-bearing entities such as capitated providers. Over half of HMOs are estimated to use nurse telephone lines and many require members to call that line before accessing other types of care (Paul 2000). Medicaid plans have also experimented with telephone triage programs in regions including Oregon and Washington, DC (Sabin 1998). Users may have different goals for a telephone triage program, but typically they seek to reduce healthcare costs and improve access to information for patients or members. By developing the ability to direct patients to the most appropriate level of care for their needs, telephone triage and decision support services offer promising tools by which risk may be managed. (See 6.1 "Telephone Triage to Reduce Out-of-Network Utilization: Kaiser Permanente" and 6.2 "Telephone Triage Overseas" at www.ache.org/pubs/mcalearney/start.cfm.)

Beyond triage, telephone-based decision support systems can also encourage self-care and promote healthy behaviors. Leveraging the value of the telephone as a tool to communicate with patients, programs incorporate telephone contact to support their tactics. Programs trying to stimulate behavior change may offer periodic telephonic nurse counseling or support as a strategy, while comprehensive programs may offer defined telephonic support in areas such as medical decision making, self-management of chronic diseases, and prenatal care (Vickery 1996).

Recent studies demonstrate substantial benefit from the use of these telephone-based population health management tools. Studies of savings attributed to the use of telephone triage systems have reported average annual savings of $50 to $240 per member user. One study conducted by vendor Access Health, Inc. along with Blue Shield of Oregon and Hewitt Associates used Medicaid claims data to compare 14,000 members with access to telephone triage services to 14,000 members without access. This study reported savings of $184 per member per year for members who had access to the triage services (Sabin 1998).

Communications Designed to Promote Self-Care

The use of communications tools to promote self-care is a demand management strategy that specifically attempts to address the notion of perceived need. Vickery and colleagues estimated that as many as one-quarter of patient visits to physicians were for conditions that these individuals could assess and treat themselves (Vickery et al. 1983). Research suggests that over three-quarters of medical care is actually self-care administered by individuals themselves (Vickery 1986; Green 1990; Vickery et al. 1988). By helping to improve an individual's ability to assess and manage his or her medical problems, self-care communications interventions are designed to educate consumers to take care of themselves. Interventions such as providing individuals with self-care books, videos, or websites have proved successful at both decreasing demand for medical care and increasing patient knowledge. Such success is also tied to cost savings. Programs providing self-care information and guidelines about care have been associated with decreases in physician visits of 7 to 17 percent (Fries et al 1993; Vickery et al. 1983). The handbook, *Take Care of Yourself* (Vickery and Fries 1994) includes many of these self-care protocols designed to help consumers address their own health needs.

In one program studying a self-care communication handbook, a large group of HMO members was given a book and medical care utilization within that group was then compared to a similar group of HMO patients who had not received the handbook. Notably, this randomized, controlled trial showed that individuals who had received the handbook made 17 percent fewer physician visits overall and 35 percent fewer visits for minor illness (Vickery et al. 1983). Similarly positive results were found using a pediatric self-care book, where the group receiving the self-care book had 14 percent fewer total visits to physicians (excluding well-baby visits). For toddlers and infants who were not firstborn, this intervention was associated with a 23-percent decrease in sick visits, 24 percent fewer phone calls to nurses for advice, and 26 percent fewer prescriptions (France, et al. 1999).

Another study designed to evaluate the effect of a health education program based on self-care communications was conducted in an HMO-based Medicare population. Using a prospective, randomized, controlled trial, researchers found a statistically significant decrease in total medical visits of 15 percent compared to the control group. This decrease in medical visits was associated with a savings of $36.65 per household (with no known negative impact on patient health). The overall program had a benefit-cost ratio of $2.19 saved for every dollar spent on program interventions (Vickery et al. 1988).

The opportunity for communications interventions to reduce inappropriate demand for medical care is one of the factors often leveraged in demand management programs. Although such communications interventions are not designed to prevent illness and disease, they can help to change individuals' knowledge of illness and perception of their need for medical care (Vickery 1996). Ideally, such changes in knowledge and beliefs can then be translated into better decisions about use of medical care services.

Information Technologies

Advances in information technology (IT) have created new avenues for delivering demand management services and interventions. Automated health assessments and Internet decision support tools are two examples of how IT can be leveraged to affect consumer demand for health and medical care services. The automation of health risk assessments and appraisals allows demand management programs to compare risk factors and the reported health status of defined populations against similar factors expected in comparable populations. When discrepancies are noted for groups or individuals, interventions can be targeted to the population to address the identified health and wellness issues. As an example, an employee population that reports a high number of smokers or a disproportionate number of individuals who note that they are in poor health can be targeted for specific behavioral interventions to address these health risk problems.

Web-based technologies can also be extremely valuable in providing demand management services, especially in delivering patient and member education. Use of the Internet in areas such as on-line health risk appraisals, on-line health resources, and on-line educational material can be successfully included in most demand management programs to enhance program effectiveness and increase patient satisfaction ("Web-based" 1997).

One healthcare system, Kaiser Permanente in Oakland, California, has reportedly developed an on-line Internet service to provide educational information, support groups, and interactive bulletin boards that facilitate question-and-answer sessions between patients and clinicians. The service was created to provide better access for members to health information, to increase flexibility in how members could access services, and to improve both communication and relationships between plan members and Kaiser doctors and staff.

The Kaiser website offers an online version of the self-care book, the *Healthwise Handbook* (Healthwise 1995), an online drug encyclopedia, and access to additional health information that is screened for quality. Members can also use the online service to request appointments or obtain advice from nurses or pharmacist educators, or to transmit messages to Kaiser staff, clinicians, or specialty physicians who will answer questions online once a week. An online health assessment provides an opportunity for Kaiser to collect information about their members, as well as give those members feedback about steps they can take to better manage their own health. Self-help discussion groups and interactive programs such as videos provide additional services for interested members. Access to the site requires a personal identification number to maintain security and confidentiality ("Use the Internet" 1997).

Cost and Clinical Effectiveness

Examples of demand management programs are found in all areas of the healthcare system. Programs developed by employers, commercial companies, providers, and the military provide examples of successful demand management strategy implementation. Program costs for demand and management typically range from $.75 to $1.25 per person per month, and many programs have demonstrated both effectiveness and cost savings (Paul 2000). However, the effectiveness and cost-effectiveness of demand management strategies is not always rigorously evaluated. Adoption or purchase of demand management tools and technologies should be accompanied by careful monitoring of population outcomes. Healthcare organizations should also take care to examine how tools were developed and for which populations such strategies were intended to serve in order to evaluate their success (Mohler and Harris 1998).

The Healthtrac Program, based on Vickery and Fries' work in the self-care area (Vickery and Fries 1994; Fries 1993), offers an example of a successful demand management program. The low-cost program is delivered by mail and is described as a computer-assisted health management program. Individuals participating in the program receive tailored recommendations and reports directing them towards specific actions to improve their health, in addition to self-care materials and newsletters. Based on large, randomized controlled trials, such programs have been associated with cost savings of 20 percent and reductions in health risks of 10 percent per year of program participation. Compared to the program's cost, savings range from 5 to 10 times the investment required (Fries 1998).

Another large study reported success with demand management for a population of Medicaid eligibles enrolled in a health maintenance organization (HMO) administered by a major insurer. The study compared eligible callers to the demand management service to eligible noncallers and noneligible Medicaid enrollees. The researchers reported that in comparison to noncallers, callers were more likely to be older, sicker, female, and have higher baseline healthcare costs. This caller group also had costs that were determined to be about 7 percent lower than noncallers. Based on these results, researchers concluded that demand management was indeed successful at improving access and long-term outcomes, including reducing costs. Further, they recommended that better outreach be targeted toward all eligibles to achieve better participation among those less likely to call for demand management services who still had higher-risk health profiles (Henderson and Hahn 1996).

Employer-based programs have also been reportedly successful. To support its employees, the Hannaford Bros. supermarket chain based in New Hampshire began offering a nurse triage line in 1993. Hannaford Bros. reported a decrease of almost 20 percent in its $20 million healthcare budget, which they attributed largely to the telephonic service (McCarthy 1997). Dow Chemical similarly reported savings associated with a telephonic decision support line implemented in 1995. Self-reports showed that 15 percent of eligible employees used the service, with more than 40 percent of callers reporting that the service helped them avoid an unnecessary physician visit and 30 percent claiming that the service had prevented at least one day lost from work (McCarthy 1997).

Dramatic savings have been similarly reported by the military, which developed a demand management program at a facility in a medically underserved rural community. Using a centralized triage concept for demand management, individuals who presented at a healthcare center without an appointment were referred to a nurse for triage. Registered nurses were used to screen and triage patients using specific protocols. Following this screening process, patients were either sent to the emergency department, received same-day appointments, or were provided with self-care education. During the initial nine months of operation, this centralized triage program processed 35,231 patients. Of these patients, 23 percent were assessed as having self-care deficits for which they received education. A 10-percent sample of these triaged and educated patients was then followed to assess their healthcare needs and satisfaction. Results of this follow-up revealed that 88 percent of these patients improved without additional intervention, and 95 percent were reportedly satisfied with the care they had received. Overall, this central triage program demonstrated annualized savings exceeding $2,500,000 based on avoidance of costs (McGraw et al. 2000).

In another example, a demand management program developed and implemented within an Army healthcare system relied on self-care interventions and a health promotion pharmacy to increase participants' health confidence, health knowledge, and practice of healthy behaviors. This program combined self-care interventions designed to manage demand and encourage appropriate use of resources, including those offered by a health promotion pharmacy. Researchers reported that the program increased participant knowledge of personal health issues and their confidence to treat minor illnesses, their practice of healthy behaviors and commitment to seek preventive services, and improved participant opinions of the healthcare system after six months of program participation. The study also found that 72 percent of the respondents (response rate of 68 percent) reported avoiding at least one visit to a healthcare clinic and 40 percent reported avoiding at least one visit to the emergency department, which was estimated as an 11:1 return on program investment (Steinweg et al. 1998).

Studies have also shown the savings potential of access to telephonic nurse counseling as part of a demand management program. In Wisconsin, the Center for Corporate Health conducted a study to test the effectiveness of a program that offered a 24-hour nurse counseling line and self-care education and included a self-care manual and newsletter. Comparing one group who had been offered only the self-care education to a second group that had also been offered access to the nurse counseling hotline, researchers found that the more extensive program saved more money per dollar invested, at $4.75 saved per dollar compared to $2.40. Similar savings were demonstrated with an Aetna counseling program, which reported savings of up to $3 per dollar invested (Goldstein 1995). (See 6.3 "Building or Buying a Demand Management Program" and 6.4 "Demand Management Companies" at www.ache.org/pubs/mcalearney/start.cfm.)

Risks of Demand Management Strategies

A definite risk of using demand management strategies is the potential for misuse of such tools. It is conceivable that, improperly used, demand management could lead to a reduction in healthcare services that is not clinically appropriate, or is not linked to improvements in clinical, economic, or humanistic outcomes. The ethical implications of utilizing such strategies must also be addressed (Malloy 1998). When programs are not supported and managed by individuals and organizations that keep patients' needs and best interests in mind, demand management recommendations may be misleading or even potentially harmful for participating patients.

People with severe problems or complex chronic diseases (e.g., multiple sclerosis) create another area of concern about the use of demand management strategies. Program administrators should be cognizant of the range of illnesses and conditions they are expected to address in the population served and specify the limitations of their services. Patients who are participating should be given sufficient information to help guide their communications with healthcare professionals to ensure that their underlying health problems are not overlooked when acute symptom management becomes a priority.

Another concern about demand management services is that such programs may inappropriately give advice or information that is specifically directive, diagnostic, or prescriptive. As Vickery notes, an important element of providing high-quality demand management services is to provide individuals with decision support rather than actual decisions (Vickery 1996). By making this distinction, programs can differentiate themselves as well as avoid potential legal problems.

Nonetheless, legal issues exist. A key distinction is made between actually making medical diagnoses and providing demand management services such as offering health information, giving advice, assessing self-reported symptoms, and triaging case seriousness. As required by law, demand management nurses cannot and do not make medical diagnoses in the process of their calls (Sullivan 1997). However, the quality of demand management services and 24-hour nurse advice lines is difficult to determine. Unless programs are housed in a managed care organization accredited by the National Committee for Quality Assurance (NCQA), such services are not reviewed nor subject to any national standards or regulations.

Healthcare attorney Gayle Sullivan (1997) has outlined a number of steps to reduce risk in demand management programs:

- Use formalized, written assessment and treatment algorithms, developed with physician input and approved by the healthcare organization.
- Review and update protocols periodically to reflect current standards of care and referral.
- Ensure use of adequately trained and experienced healthcare professionals.
- Do not include pay bonuses for nurses based on the number of calls or on the cost-saving advice that they dispense.
- Have both primary care physicians and specialists involved and available to help nurses and other providers who answer calls.
- Institute a formal quality improvement program for the demand management service including concurrent call monitoring, recording and analyzing calls, reviewing clinical situations, periodic testing and training of staff, and regular patient follow-up.

A final concern about many demand management programs is that the underlying goal of such strategies may seem to be cost reduction instead of guiding appropriate medical care use. This concern, however, is rarely warranted. Instead, as noted by Vickery (1996), self-interested individuals who are supported by demand management services end up using fewer and less costly services for three reasons:

1. These individuals live healthy lifestyles and thus have fewer preventable illnesses and lower morbidity.
2. Through demand management programs, these individuals have access to decision and behavior support services that help increase confidence in their ability to assess and manage their own medical problems, thereby reducing their perceived need for medical care.
3. Such individuals who are participating in medical decision making with their physicians have increased knowledge of treatment risks

and benefits and ultimately tend to choose less risky and less expensive treatments because of their inherent risk aversion.

This combination of factors supports the idea that effective demand management services that educate and empower consumers can reduce costs and inappropriate medical care utilization by helping consumers make better healthcare decisions.

Benefits of Demand Management Strategies

Demand management programs reportedly receive very positive support from users of such services. Patients appreciate having access to healthcare professionals while being provided with opportunities to increase personal knowledge about their own health conditions. Healthcare organizations report savings associated with more appropriate utilization and increased patient satisfaction. Finally, employers value such programs because they save money and improve employee health and well-being.

Benefits to Patients

One major benefit to patients who participate in demand management programs is derived from patient education. Research has shown that patients who receive education about communicating with physicians prior to visits ask more appropriate and succinct questions and these questions can be answered with specific information for that patient (McGee and Cegala 1998; Cegala et al. 2001). As empowerment is increased through education and communications about self-care options, consumers become both better informed and more self-confident in their abilities to make decisions about treatment options. This increased confidence is associated with feelings of greater self-efficacy as consumers become less dependent on medical care services and more apt to practice healthy behaviors and improve their quality of life (O'Leary 1985; Montrose 1995).

Another potential benefit for patients is that demand management programs can help consumers meet or exceed their expectations for care. Patients' expectations for medical care come from multiple sources, can be very complex, and are not always met. A study of unmet expectations for care by Kravitz et al. (1996) reported that issues such as the patient's current somatic symptoms, his or her perceived vulnerability to illness, past experiences with similar illnesses, and patient knowledge acquired from physicians, friends, family, or the media could all shape patients' perceptions and expectations for care. In the context of demand management, these factors are similar to the different components Vickery noted as affecting demand, especially morbidity, perceived need, and patient preferences. Demand management programs can benefit patients by shaping their understanding of medical conditions and their perceptions about needed medical care. By attempting to educate individuals using a demand management framework, programs can help patients be better informed and can responsibly influence these patients to make appropriate medical care decisions. In addition, it becomes more likely that these patients' expectations for care will be met.

The fact that patients occasionally demand inappropriate or unnecessary care, knowingly or unknowingly, is well-documented. Parents may demand antibiotics for their children when the etiologic origin of the disease is viral, and women may request cesareans for normal births for a variety of reasons. End-of-life issues create another area where services are demanded to provide medical care in situations where such care is either deemed unproven or even futile. Many physicians are willing to provide such services, given that care is part of the patient's wishes and all insurance coverage issues are resolvable (Friedman 1996). Although advance directives for medical care are recommended to properly record patients' wishes about life-sustaining treatments, actual use is infrequent (Emanuel et al. 1991). Demand management programs can aid both patients and physicians in circumstances where demands for medical care may not be appropriate and where alternatives such as counseling, support, and education can help.

Yet another benefit patients can derive from demand management programs is help negotiating the complex healthcare system. Demand management services may include elements such as facilitating direct access to specialists or referrals to emergency departments ("Patients Reap" 1998). Demand management programs can also serve as an entry point to more involved chronic disease management by using outbound calls to assess patients and stratify them for referral to disease management programs. By serving as a point of access to a provider or healthcare system, a demand management program can help allay patient concerns about seeking care as well as direct patients to the most appropriate providers.

Benefits to Healthcare Organizations and Providers

Healthcare organizations and individual providers may also benefit from demand management programs. With better informed and educated patients, organizations at risk for the cost of care for their members may save money by achieving more appropriate medical care utilization. Even in shared risk arrangements, programs that provide consumers with information about appropriate demand for services can help decrease expenses associated with nonmedical reasons for seeking care or expenses attributable to individuals who seek care at an inappropriate level of intensity.

Another benefit of more educated and informed consumers is that such patients are less inclined to make malpractice claims against their providers. With effective communication and increases in patient satisfaction, the risk of malpractice claims is reduced for both physicians and healthcare institutions (Lester and Smith 1993).

From the physician standpoint, providers may appreciate increased health knowledge among patients who are less inclined to demand unnecessary and time-consuming visits. Given the time constraints on physicians' schedules, having help from a demand management program that will provide necessary education supports clinical goals for patient education. Education provided through demand management programs may also help patients become more informed consumers and enable them to make more efficient use of provider time when they do seek medical care in person (Cegala et al. 2001). Furthermore, such education about communications with providers has been demonstrated to improve patient compliance with suggested treatment regimens (Cegala et al. 2000), providing another tangible benefit for both providers and patients.

Benefits to Employers

Employers who sponsor demand management programs clearly benefit from providing these services. According to Fronstin (1996) of the Employee Benefits Research Institute (EBRI), many employers attempt to contain healthcare costs by using demand management programs. A survey of major employers found that 88 percent had introduced some program involving health promotion, disease prevention, or early intervention designed to encourage healthy lifestyles among salaried employees (Fronstin 1996). Employer benefits of work-sponsored demand management programs include increased productivity, employee retention, and improved employee morale demonstrated by reductions in employee turnover and absenteeism. With these benefits easily tied to financial savings, employers remain very interested in the potential of demand management strategies.

Conclusion

Ideally, a demand management strategy is designed to extend the reach of healthcare institutions and providers in a formal framework. Triage centers, nurse counselors, and other demand management personnel can supplement available medical care services by providing 24-hour access to guided advice and decision support. High-quality demand management programs can be viewed as an added benefit for both patients and physicians who are associated with the health plans, employers, and providers who offer their services. Leveraging this value can be a key success factor for an institution that is trying to promote itself as being responsive to consumer demands and sensitive to consumer needs.

As this chapter has shown, demand management strategies offer the potential to reduce and improve demand for medical care, and this is appealing to both patients and payers. By using strategies such as telephone triage and decision support and communications designed to promote self-care, demand management programs can address issues such as morbidity, perceived need, and patient preferences for medical care. When delivered effectively to a defined population, demand management strategies have the potential to both improve the quality of care and reduce medical costs by helping consumers make informed decisions about appropriate use of the healthcare system.

REFERENCES

Anders, G. 1997. "Telephone Triage." *The Wall Street Journal* (February 4): A1, A6.

Andersen, R., and J. F. Newman. 1973. "Societal and Individual Determinants of Medical Care Utilization in the United States." *Milbank Quarterly* 51 (1): 95–121.

Berkanovic, E., C. Telesky, and S. Reeder. 1981. "Structural and Social Psychological Factors in the Decision to Seek Medical Care for Symptoms." *Medical Care* 19 (7): 693–709.

Cegala, D. J., T. Marinelli, and D. M. Post. 2000. "The Effects of Patient Communication Skills Training on Compliance." *Archives of Family Medicine* 9 (1): 57–64.

Cegala, D. J., D. M. Post, and L. M. McClure. 2001. "The Effect of Patient Communication Skills Training on the Discourse of Elderly Patients During a Primary Care Interview." *Journal of the American Geriatrics Society* 49 (11): 1505–11.

Connelly, J. E., J. T. Philbrick, G. R. Smith, Jr., D. L. Kaiser, and A. Wymer. 1989. "Health Perceptions of Primary Care Patients and the Influence on Healthcare Utilization." *Medical Care* 27 (supplement): S99–S109.

Connelly, J. E., G. R. Smith, Jr., J. T. Philbrick, and D. L. Kaiser. 1991. "Healthy Patients Who Perceive Poor Health and Their Use of Primary Care Services." *Journal of General Internal Medicine* 6 (1): 47–51.

Emanuel, L. L., M. J. Barry, J. D. Stoeckle, L. M. Ettelson, and E. J. Emanuel. 1991. "Advance Directives for Medical Care: A Case for Greater Use." *New England Journal of Medicine* 324 (13): 889–95.

France, E. K., M. J. Selna, E. E. Lyons, A. L. Beck, and B. N. Calonge. 1999. "Effect of a Pediatric Self-care Book on Utilization of Services in a Group Model HMO." *Clinical Pediatrics* 38 (12): 709–15.

Friedman, E. 1996. "Making Choices." *Healthcare Forum Journal* 3 (31): 11.

Fries, J. F. 1993. *Living Well*. Reading, MA: Addison-Wesley Publishing Co.

Fries, J. F. 1998. "Reducing the Need and Demand for Medical Services." *Psychosomatic Medicine* 60 (2): 140–42.

Fries, J. F., C. E. Koop, C. E. Beadle, P. P. Cooper, M. J. England, R. F. Greaves, J. J. Sokolov, and D. Wright. 1993. "Reducing Healthcare Costs by Reducing the Need and Demand for Medical Services." *New England Journal of Medicine* 329 (5): 321–25.

Fronstin, P. 1996. "Health Promotion and Disease Prevention: A Look at Demand Management Programs." *EBRI Issue Brief* (Sep.) 177: 1–14.

Goldstein, M. A. 1995. "Demand Management Looks Promising, Too." *Modern Healthcare* (August 21): 144.

Green, K. E. 1990. "Common Illnesses and Self-care" *Journal of Community Health* 15 (5): 329–38.

Healthwise, Inc. 1995. *Healthwise Handbook,* 12th ed. Boise, ID: Healthwise, Inc.

Henderson, M. G., and W. M. Hahn. 1996. "Can Demand Management Programs Increase Access to Care While Controlling Costs?" [Abstract], AHSR and FHSR Abstract Book, 13: 31.

Kaplan, G., and T. Camacho. 1983. "Perceived Health and Mortality: A Nine-year Follow-up of the Human Population Laboratory Cohort." *American Journal of Epidemiology* 117 (3): 292–304.

Kravitz, R. L., E. J. Callahan, D. Paterniti, D. Antonius, M. Dunham, and C. E. Lewis. 1996. "Prevalence and Sources of Patients' Unmet Expectations for Care." *Annals of Internal Medicine* 125 (9): 730–37.

Lester, G. W., and S. G. Smith. 1993. "Listening and Talking to Patients: A Remedy for Malpractice Suits?" *Western Journal of Medicine* 158 (3): 268–72.

Lynch, W. D., D. W. Edington, and A. Johnson. 1996. "Predicting the Demand for Healthcare." *Healthcare Forum Journal* 39 (1): 20–24.

MacStravic, S. 1996. "Managing Utilization: The Old Way and the New Way." *Health Care Strategic Management* 14 (10): 1: 20–21.

MacStravic, S., and G. Montrose. 1998. *Managing Health Care Demand.* Gaithersberg, MD: Aspen Publishers.

Malloy, C. 1998. "Managed Care and Ethical Implications in Telephone-based Health Services." *Advanced Practice Nursing Quarterly* 4 (2): 30–33.

Marosits, M. J.1997. "Improving Financial and Patient Outcomes: the Future of Demand Management." *Healthcare Financial Management* 51 (8): 43–44.

McCarthy, R. 1997. "It Takes More than a Phone Call to Manage Demand." *Business and Health* 15 (5): 36–41.

McGee, D. S., and D. J. Cegala. 1998. "Patient Communication Skills Training for Improved Communication Competence in Primary Care Medical Consultation." *Journal of Applied Communication Research* 26 (4): 412–30.

McGinnis, J. M., and W. H. Foege. 1993. "Actual Causes of Death in the United States." *Journal of the American Medical Association* 270 (18): 2207–12.

McGraw, E., H. Barthel, and M. Arrington. 2000. "A Model for Demand Management in a Managed Care Environment." *Military Medicine* 165 (4): 305–8.

Mohler, M. J., and J. M. Harris, Jr. 1998. "Demand Management: Another Marketing Tool or a Way to Quality Care? *Journal of Evaluation in Clinical Practice* 4 (2): 103–11.

Montrose, G. 1995. "Demand Management May Help Stem Costs." *Health Management Technology* 16 (2): 18–21.

Newhouse, J. P. 1994. *Free for All: Lessons from the Rand Health Insurance Experiment.* Cambridge, MA: Harvard University Press.

O'Leary, A. 1985. "Self-efficacy and Health." *Behavior Research Therapy* 23 (4): 437–51.

"Patients Reap the Benefits of Demand Management." 1998. *Physician Relations Update* (Feb): 14–16.

Paul, K. A. 2000. "Managing the Demand for Health Services by Adopting Patient-centered Programs." *Benefits Quarterly* (Second Quarter): 54–59.

Sabin, M. 1998. "Telephone Triage Improves Demand Management Effectiveness." *Healthcare Financial Management* 52 (8): 49–51.

Steinweg, K. K., R. E. Killingsworth, R. J. Nannini, and J. Spayde. 1998. "The Impact on a Healthcare System of a Program to Facilitate Self-care." *Military Medicine* 163 (3): 139–44.

Sullivan, G. 1997. "Advice or Diagnosis? A Legal Perspective." *Business and Health* 15, (5): 40–42.

Tanner, J. L., W. C. Cockerham, and J. L. Speth . 1983. "Predicting Physician Utilization." *Medical Care* 21 (3): 360–69.

"Use the Internet to Reach More Patients with your Demand Management Programs." 1997. *Healthcare Demand and Disease Management* 3 (5): 75–77.

Vickery, D. M. 1986. "Medical Self-care: A Review of the Concept and Program Models." *American Journal of Health Promotion* 1 (1): 23–28.

Vickery, D. M. 1996. "Toward Appropriate Use of Medical Care." *Healthcare Forum Journal* 39 (1): 15–19.

Vickery, D. M., H. Kalmer, D. Lowry, M. Constantine, E. Wright, and W. Loren. 1983. "Effect of a Self-care Education Program on Medical Visits." *Journal of the American Medical Association* 250 (21): 2952–56.

Vickery, D. M., and J. F. Fries. 1994. *Take Care of Yourself—A Consumer's Guide to Medical Care,* 3rd ed. Reading, MA: Addison-Wesley Publishing Co.

Vickery, D. M., T. J. Golaszewski, E. C. Wright, and H. Kalmer. 1988. "The Effect of Self-care Interventions on the Use of Medical Service Within a Medicare Population." *Medical Care* 26 (6): 580–88.

Vickery, D. M., H. Kalmer, D. Lowry, M. Constantine, E. Wright, and W. Loren. 1983. "Effect of a Self-care Education Program on Medical Visits." *Journal of the American Medical Association* 250 (21): 2952–56.

Vickery, D. M., and W. D. Lynch. 1995. "Demand Management: Enabling Patients to Use Medical Care Appropriately." *Journal of Occupational and Environmental Medicine* 37 (5): 551–57.

"Web-based Patient Education Becoming a Powerful Tool in Demand Management." 1997. *Healthcare Demand and Disease Management* 3 (9): 138–40.

DISEASE MANAGEMENT

Disease management strategies use health status criteria to define the population. While many definitions of disease management have been circulated, optimistic versions see disease management as a strategy that moves beyond cost-control goals to improve population health and individual health outcomes. Defined as "a systematic, population-based approach to identify persons at risk, intervene with a specific program of care, and measure clinical and other outcomes" (Epstein 1996; Bodenheimer 1999), disease management strategies have gained popularity as these programs meet their promises to reduce healthcare costs while improving or maintaining quality of care and service.

Definition

The following is the formal definition of disease management set forth by the Disease Management Association of America (DMAA 2002): "Disease management is a system of coordinated healthcare interventions and communications for populations with conditions in which patient self-care efforts are significant. Disease management:

- supports the physician- or practitioner-patient relationship and plan of care;
- emphasizes prevention of exacerbations and complications utilizing evidence-based practice guidelines and patient empowerment strategies; and
- evaluates clinical, humanistic, and economic outcomes on an ongoing basis with the goal of improving overall health."

The Association further states that disease management should contain "population identification processes; evidence-based practice guidelines; collaborative practice models to include physician and support service providers; patient self-management education; process and outcomes measurement, evaluation, and management; and routine reporting/feedback loops (DMAA 2002). Designing and implementing disease management programs that contain these components clearly benefits both patients and payers with an integrated and outcomes-based focus.

The distinction between illness-focused disease management and individual, case-focused conventional case management is best described as a contrast between more and less comprehensive care management strategies.

Overall, disease management benefits from a comprehensive, integrated approach rarely emphasized in traditional case management. Emphasizing health management, education, and prevention of progression of diseases, disease management attempts to improve long-term outcomes for patients along the continuum of care instead of merely concentrating on cost control for expensive patients (Plocher 1997).

A key component of current disease management programs is the importance of coordinating services for the population of individuals served. Ellrodt and colleagues (1997) emphasize this in their description that notes, "disease management is an approach to patient care that coordinates medical resources for patients across the entire healthcare delivery system." By being both broad and coordinated, disease management strategies in population health management can span different types of data and providers and can improve financial, clinical, and functional outcomes.

Burden of Chronic Illness

As described in Chapter 1, the burden of chronic illness in the United States is substantial in both human and economic terms. With nearly half of all Americans living with at least one chronic condition and an estimated $510 billion in direct medical costs associated with care for chronic conditions in 2000 (Partnership for Solutions 2001), the need to address this problem is clear. Disease management strategies that attempt to improve the quality of care for persons with chronic illness hold interest for most entities that bear financial risk for the cost of caring for such illnesses. Table 7.1 compares the prevalence, incidence, and costs of selected chronic diseases in the United States.

In practice, three of the top contributors to medical care utilization and healthcare costs are key candidates for disease management programs: congestive heart failure, diabetes mellitus, and asthma. *Heart disease* is actually the leading cause of illness-related mortality in the United States. According to 1997 statistics, almost 60 million Americans suffer from one or more forms of cardiac disease. Specifically, coronary heart disease affects over 12 million persons, with 7.7 million having had a myocardial infarction and 4.4 million having suffered a stroke. Cardiac diseases were responsible for 41.2 percent of all deaths in the United States in 1997, claiming almost 1 million lives. Coronary heart disease alone ranks first among causes of death for Americans. Annually, it is estimated that 1.25 million persons experience a heart attack, and the mortality rate from these heart attacks is 40 percent (American Heart Association 2001; AHCPR 1999).

Given the prevalence of heart disease in the United States, it is no surprise that the economic cost of heart disease is staggering. It is estimated that 7.9 percent of the $203 billion spent on Medicare in 1995 was attributed to ischemic heart disease. Utilization figures are also alarming.

Disease	Prevalence in 1994 (millions)	Incidence in 1994 (per 1000)	Total Costs in 1997 Dollars ($U.S. billions)
Heart disease	22.3	85.8	167.2
Cancer	7.4–8.1[a]	4.1	104.0
Diabetes	7.7	29.8	98.2
Arthritis	33.4	128.8	83.5[b]
Bronchitis	14.0	54.0	28.7[b]
Influenza	90.4	348.0	17.5[b]
Asthma	14.6	56.1	15.1[b]

TABLE 7.1
Prevalence, Incidence, and Total Costs of Selected Chronic Diseases in the United States

[a] Estimated prevalence, 1997.
[b] U.S. Bureau of Labor Statistics: Percentage change in medical care consumer price index, U.S. 1987 to U.S. 1997.
SOURCE: Adapted from Musich, S. A., W. N. Burton, and D. W. Edington. 1999. "Costs and Benefits of Prevention and Disease Management." *Disease Management and Health Outcomes* 5 (3): 153–66. Reported in "California Law Poses Serious Threat to DM Programs." 1999. *Healthcare Demand and Disease Management* (Oct.): 153–55.

In the United States in 1995 it was estimated that cardiac diseases were responsible for 573,000 coronary artery bypass grafts (CABG) at a cost of $44,820 each and 4,000 angioplasties at an average cost of $20,370. Similarly, approximately 3.2 million ambulatory care visits and 926,000 hospital discharges in 1995 were attributable to cerebrovascular disease. Such utilization was associated with an average hospital cost for stroke from admission to discharge of $18,244 per person under age 65 (AHCPR 1999).

Diabetes is a chronic illness that has no cure and is the seventh leading cause of death in the United States. Almost 6 percent of adults or 15.7 million people are afflicted with diabetes mellitus. Unfortunately, only 10.3 million of these people have been diagnosed with diabetes while 5.4 million persons are not aware they have the disease. Diabetes is the leading cause of new cases of blindness in the 20 to 74 year old population and the leading cause of limb loss. Furthermore, diabetics are 2 to 4 times more likely to have heart disease and 2 to 4 times more likely to suffer a stroke than nondiabetics.

According to the American Diabetes Association, the total economic cost of diabetes in the United States was $98 billion in 1997. Specifically, direct medical and treatment costs resulting from treating patients with diabetes are calculated to be approximately $44 billion per year. Employers are estimated to pay another $54 billion annually in indirect costs resulting from absenteeism, disability, lost productivity, and premature death (American Diabetes Association 2002). Utilization figures are similarly distressing. Diabetes was responsible for over 3 million hospital days and 15.6 million ambulatory care visits in 1995 alone (AHCPR 1999).

Asthma statistics are no less stark. In the United States, asthma affects an even greater proportion of the population than coronary heart disease or diabetes, afflicting more than 14 million Americans. Estimates from 1994 reported that asthma was associated with $7.8 billion in annual total costs, including $5.1 billion estimated for direct medical care expenditures such as ambulatory care visits, hospital outpatient and inpatient services, visits to the emergency department, physician fees, and prescription medications. Over half of the direct costs (56 percent) attributable to asthma are estimated to be associated with patient hospitalizations and could potentially be reduced if asthma was better managed (Gillespie 1999). Additional concern about asthma stems from the fact that its prevalence is increasing in the American population without a clear understanding of the reasons why. The mortality and morbidity associated with asthma are also increasing, most notably higher among low-income and minority groups (Gillespie 1999).

Given this substantial burden from chronic illnesses in the U.S., it is no surprise that disease management programs have emerged to attempt to better manage the problems and costs associated with these illnesses. Program components such as patient education, chronic disease management, care coordination, and quality and outcomes improvement are seen as critical for successful disease management efforts.

Such programs that approach chronic illness with an eye towards enabling patients to manage their own illnesses can help both improve clinical outcomes and patient health as well as reduce utilization.

The Context of Disease Management

The question of how to distinguish disease management from other medical management strategies is both philosophical and practical. From a population health management perspective, disease management is important because it focuses on a distinct population, defined by disease. Rather than considering individual patients on a case-by-case basis or focus on utilization patterns in the acute care setting, disease management uses a population-based approach to care that crosses all settings.

Depending on perspective, the term disease management can encompass a number of different program models: (1) single illness chronic disease management programs; (2) single illness programs targeted towards rare or catastrophic diseases; and (3) comprehensive approaches with titles such as care management, care coordination, or total health management programs. Recognizing that all of these approaches can be classified as disease management programs, for the purposes of this book, each of these models will be discussed separately in different chapters. This chapter will focus on chronic disease management programs typically developed around

one disease, while Chapter 8 describes catastrophic care management programs, and Chapter 10 focuses on a comprehensive approach to integrating population health management strategies.

Using a disease management model, care processes are monitored
and measured together in a systems-focused approach to care instead of relying on the individual clinical activities of different providers (Todd and Nash
1997). Multidisciplinary teams of providers must strive for good communication as they work together to provide coordinated healthcare services.
Disease management is also very consistent with a quality improvement
model. When programs are outcomes-focused and take continuous quality
improvement (CQI) principles into consideration, they have great potential to improve multiple outcomes including clinical, behavioral, and cost.

The characteristics of a disease management strategy tend to reflect
a continuous improvement process: standards of care are set; protocols can
be developed and implemented to achieve goals to meet those standards;
outcomes are measured; and systems of care are improved (Joshi and Bernard
1999). This process helps a disease management strategy include multiple
factors that are consistent with CQI principles:

1. Commitment to quality
2. Focus on the patient
3. Use of multidisciplinary teams
4. Data-driven approach;
5. Application of performance measurement systems
6. Integrated and aligned management

Disease Management Industry

The term disease management is attributed to a report developed by the
Boston Consulting Group in 1995 describing a project done in the pharmaceutical industry. Current disease management programs are designed
to help healthcare organizations focus on a defined population of individuals who are in need of coordinated care and interventions. These programs have emerged under the sponsorship of many different types of entities and each of these players has had varying degrees of success with program
development and implementation as the industry has evolved. Disease management program sponsors fall under seven general headings, and these
are each discussed below.

Pharmaceutical firms and Pharmacy Benefits Managers (PBMs)

Initially, pharmaceutical firms and PBMs took the lead in working with
health plans to develop disease-specific programs. From the origin of the
term to much of the stigma associated with disease management as an
opportunity for pharmaceutical firms to push their particular drugs, the
pharmaceutical industry can be given a substantial amount of credit for the
development of the disease management approach.

PBMs often provide disease management programs directly to employers or managed care organizations in the context of general benefit management services (Gillespie 1999; Novartis 1998). A 1998 report from Novartis reported that 75 percent of all pharmacy directors in PBMs had identified expenditures associated with the development of disease management programs. Further, HMOs noted that 16 percent of their disease management programs were provided through PBMs (Gillespie 1999), with many of these programs developed specifically for diseases that either respond to or rely upon pharmaceutical products or services. In 1997, the five most common disease management program initiatives by PBMs included asthma, gastrointestinal disorders, diabetes, hypertension, and dyslipidemia (Novartis 1998). Although the PBMs and pharmaceutical firms tend to be responsible for a smaller proportion of the current disease management business, they remain active in their participation (Ritterband 2000). (See 7.1 "Pharmacists and Disease Management" at www.ache.org/pubs/mcalearney/start.cfm.)

Managed Care Organizations (MCOs)

Due to both their mission to improve quality while controlling costs and their financial situation in assuming risk for capitated lives, the interest of MCOs in this population health management approach is no surprise. A 1998 report from the Boston Consulting Group reported that 76 percent of pharmacy directors from HMOs had some sort of disease management program for their members (Gillespie 1999), whether developed in-house or outsourced to a PBM or vendor.

For most MCOs, disease management programs are actually very consistent with their medical management approach. CIGNA HealthCare's asthma program reportedly helped both patients and physicians by avoiding complications that would require hospitalizations and encouraging appropriate use of medications. In 1997, their program showed a 23-percent reduction in admissions to hospitals and an improvement of 15 percent in use of medications. Similarly, a congestive heart failure program initiated by United HealthCare of Northeast Ohio has shown reductions in hospitalizations and overall hospital days (Gillespie 1999).

Health Services and Provider Organizations

Especially when they are at risk for the medical care expenses of their patients, health services and provider organizations also have an interest in sponsoring disease management programs. Depending on the size of the organization and the type of contracts they maintain with MCOs and other insurers, providers have varying degrees of interest. When provider organizations are small or if they do not have a strong information systems capability, such providers may choose to work with other sponsors to support a disease management program. However, when such an organization has the capability to identify and stratify patients, as well as to measure and monitor clinical and financial outcomes, such organizations emerge as another strong sponsor of disease management strategies.

Because health services organizations such as integrated delivery systems or major hospital systems are typically large enough to support the types of data monitoring and outcomes measurement necessary for disease management programs, they can be ideal settings for disease management. Product lines have emerged in these provider institutions to support organization of care services around particular disease entities and treatment patterns. Very important in these provider and health services organizations is the organizational commitment to disease management as a health and quality of care improvement approach. With leadership commitment and clinician involvement in the design, development, and implementation of disease management approaches, such healthcare entities have emerged as successful proponents and users of disease management strategies.

Employers

Employers are also interested in sponsoring disease management programs, especially when they can bring a return on their investment. A 1997 survey completed by the National Managed Health Care Congress and Migliara/Kaplan Associates reported that 19 percent of employer respondents would implement a disease management program if the program savings matched the program cost, while another 29 percent required a 5 to 10 percent savings expectation. Further employer data showed that 46 percent of employers were interested in developing a disease management program specifically to decrease their total costs, while another 30 percent stated that making their workforce healthier was their primary concern ("Employers" 1998).

Disease management programs are especially interesting to employers when they can be targeted towards diseases associated with high levels of absenteeism and reductions in productivity. This employer interest recognizes the burden of chronic illness on employers who lose money when employees suffer from poor health. The 1997 survey ("Employers" 1998) found that employers had particular interest in disease management programs when they could be designed to help manage long- and short-term disability claims and to help manage the costs of workers' compensation. (This strategy is discussed further in Chapter 9.)

Although employers are infrequently interested in developing and running their own disease management programs in-house, a variety of contracts with vendors and pharmacy benefits managers have emerged for employer-based initiatives. The same 1997 survey revealed that the most current and future interest in disease management programs was to offer programs through the employer's general health contractor. However, the survey also showed a considerable growing interest in carving out disease management services to a specific disease management provider, on either a fee-for-service or capitated basis ("Employers" 1998).

Behavioral Health Providers

Providers such as managed behavioral health organizations represent another group with interest in disease management opportunities. While behavioral health disease management has not been developed as a specialty carve-out, it can be argued that the disease management model is very appropriate. As described by Jay Pomerantz (2000), focusing on improving outcomes and reducing costs for schizophrenic, manic depressive, major depressive, and panic disorder patients within the defined population of health plan or behavioral health plan members may be very effective. Clinical measures including depression scores on standardized tests, compliance with medication regimens, and use of medical disability can all be evaluated. Decreasing expenditures for unnecessary x-rays, ECGs, and MRIs for panic disorder patients; improving smoking cessation results; and reducing problems associated with substance abuse represent reasonable targets for such programs (Pomerantz 2000). Considering behavioral health issues in the context of either disease management or disability management can improve the effectiveness of both types of strategies as health and well-being are maximized.

Medicaid Agencies

Medicaid agencies in different states have been another sponsor of disease management initiatives, due largely to their increased interest in reducing healthcare program costs and developing more comprehensive health management approaches. At this point, almost half of the states in the U.S. offer disease management programs—through their Medicaid agencies, and they are most commonly focused on asthma, diabetes, or congestive heart failure (Gillespie 1999).

Using the defined Medicaid population, innovative approaches to disease management have also been developed. Programs addressing sickle cell anemia, HIV/AIDs, and high-risk pregnancies have all shown success in both improving health and reducing costs among the Medicaid population (Rabinowitz 2001). Programs that expand the disease management model to address overall health and well-being issues have also proved effective. A program in Milwaukee for children with special needs reported improvements in both clinical and functional outcomes as well as reductions in juvenile offenses and utilization of residential treatment ("Two Managed" 2001). Similarly, a Kentucky program designed to increase participation in the early periodic screening, diagnosis, and treatment (EPSDT) program reported increases in well-child visits to almost 50 percent, and achievement of additional outcomes exceeding the mean for Medicaid in 97 percent of their measures (Rabinowitz 2001).

State-wide Medicaid disease management programs show encouraging results. The managed Medicaid demonstration program in North Carolina initially developed an asthma management program and then, inspired by its success, included a diabetes management program as well ("Two Medicaid" 2001). The current programs cover about 14 percent of the population with asthma and 7 percent with diabetes in the demonstration sites. To pay for the program, $2.50 per member per month is provided by the state to cover the costs of care management and other program expenses. Program effectiveness is assessed by a review of performance measures such as keeping diabetic flow charts in the medical records and having patients make continued care visits at least twice per year, as well as outcome measures such as hospital admissions and emergency room visits for diabetic complications. State data have provided support to develop more disease management initiatives in areas such as otitis media, gastroenteristis, and high-risk pregnancy. (See 7.2 "Medicaid Disease Management in Pennsylvania" at www.ache.org/pubs/mcalearney/start.cfm.)

Independent vendors represent the fastest growing sector of the disease management industry. Currently, over 150 companies offer some version of a disease management program, and overall industry revenues exceeded $350 million in 1999. Vendors allow program sponsors to outsource all or parts of their disease management programs, depending on the level of service needed. Programs offered range from little more than written protocols and guidelines with online information to comprehensive disease management programs that guarantee cost savings. Depending on the needs and goals of the program sponsor, vendors can tailor projects and programs to meet multiple objectives. Several vendors have developed very good reputations within the industry and offer disease management programs with a savings guarantee. This type of financial arrangement can be very attractive to the sponsoring entity that needs to show proof of program value to obtain resources for program development.

Independent Vendors

Organization in the Industry

The Disease Management Purchasing Consortium and Advisory Council (DMPC) represents a group of 48 health plans concerned about disease management activities. Founded by Alfred Lewis (who also organized the nonprofit Disease Management Association of America), the Consortium provides contracting assistance to health plans interested in pursuing disease management initiatives. The Consortium strives to help its full members (health plans, employers, and physician groups) by providing contracting assistance in the disease management field. Their website (www.dismgmt.com) reports that, defined by dollar volume, the Consortium has been involved in around 70 percent of all outsourced disease and population management programs that have been contracted or implemented as of 2001.

In addition to full members, the Consortium also serves as an organizing body for associate members including vendors, venture capital firms, consulting firms, academic medical centers, trade associations, regulatory and governmental bodies, and executive recruiters, all of whom are interested in the disease and population management industry. The Consortium offers access to information and conferences related to disease management and tries to centralize educational and strategic information about disease management program provision.

The use of multiple vendors in the disease management area has led to considerable variability in service. To reduce some of this variability, the Disease Management Association of America (www.dmaa.org) was founded in March of 1999. This nonprofit, voluntary organization represents both health plans and disease management companies. Its mission is to advance the field of disease management by promoting high-quality standards and educating physicians, consumers, payers, accreditation bodies, and legislators about the potential value of disease management in enhancing individual and population-based health.

Regulatory Issues

As with many new business opportunities, disease management initiatives have attracted the attention of regulatory bodies concerned with maintaining good quality of care and service for patients and providers. This regulatory interest may impact disease management program development as it affects reimbursement, provider participation, or even program scope.

In California, the governor has recently signed legislation prohibiting disease management programs from treating patients without approval from physicians ("Prevention" 1999). Similarly, a different measure was passed requiring health professionals who provide medical advice services to any patients residing in the State of California to be licensed in the state by the end of 2000 (Barnett et al. 1999). Because regulatory requirements such as these are very restrictive to disease management companies, they may affect both vendor and health plan willingness to contract for services in different locations. Continued monitoring of these regulatory trends will be critical for the disease management industry.

Accreditation Issues

In response to the tremendous growth in disease management, the National Committee for Quality Assurance (NCQA) issued standards for a new Disease Management Accreditation and Certification program in December 2001. The NCQA offers three accreditation programs to review disease management functions, depending on whether the entity is focused on providing services to patients, practitioners, or both. The standards for accreditation have been defined through the NCQA process using an independent, outside review to ensure rigor and relevance. A certification program is also available with three options: program design certification, systems certification, and contact certification. The certification programs attempt to evaluate the effectiveness of the disease management organization in providing patient outreach, designing clinical information systems, and developing educational materials related to disease management.

Twenty organizations have adopted the NCQA programs, including health plans, pharmaceutical firms, and independent vendors. Managed care organizations, managed behavioral health organizations, and preferred provider organizations contracting with disease management organizations who are certified will receive credit towards their own accreditation on NCQA quality improvement standards. Ideally, the accreditation and certification processes are designed to help identify organizations who can provide disease management services that effectively improve health outcomes for individuals and populations who are seriously or chronically ill (NCQA 2001).

Disease Management Historical Developments

One means of classifying disease management programs is by generations. This model was developed by Gervitz et al. (1999) and describes three generations of disease management program development that focus on program content. The first generation of disease management programs was developed by the pharmaceutical industry to increase market share and was characterized by mass mailings for patient education, limited use of clinical guidelines, and mailings to providers describing current disease treatment standards. Patient outcomes were not measured, and treatment appropriateness was not emphasized. A disease-focused approach was believed to increase the effectiveness of drug therapies in practice, promote a particular pharmaceutical regimen, and reduce medical care costs for the health plan or insurance company sponsoring the disease management program. Not surprisingly, many health plans reacted unfavorably to such tactics to push particular drugs and rejected the notion of disease management approaches because of their pharmaceutical firm origins. (See 7.3 "Phases in Demand Management Program Development at www.ache.org/pubs/mcalearney/start.cfm.)

Second generation programs used the 80:20 rule in healthcare to focus on the sickest 20 percent of the patients who typically account for 80 percent of health plan's total costs. Focusing on these patients, disease management programs were developed that captured immediate savings through an intensive case management approach (Gervitz et al. 1999).

The third generation of disease management programs expanded organizations' perspectives to consider the needs of a greater population of patients. By trying to integrate patient care across a continuum of services, these programs attempted to provide a true population health management approach. Such programs typically leverage the benefits of early detection of problems and use sophisticated information systems to aid the management process. Using this third generation model, monitoring patient progress is fundamental to the program and outcomes assessment is critical (Gervitz et al. 1999).

Disease management strategies have found their place in the American healthcare system. Whether offered by vendors, health plans, or medical

FIGURE 7.1
Percent of All
Care that Will
Be Subject to
Disease
Management

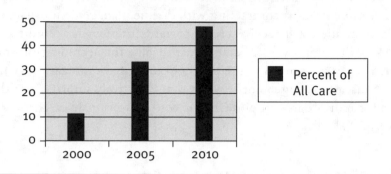

SOURCE: Institute for the Future; modified from Scott, L. 1999. "It's All in the Delivery; Disease
Management: The Right Care at the Right Time." *Modern Physician* (September) 1: 30–40.

groups, the percentage of healthcare subject to disease management is
expected to grow in the coming years. As shown in Figure 7.1, projections
from the Institute for the Future show disease management growing from
affecting around 10 percent of all care in 2000 to as much as half of the
care offered by some organizations. Figure 7.2 shows the percentage of
care for six conditions projected to be subject to disease management. Over
70 percent of the care for these six conditions (diabetes, CHF, COPD,
asthma, cancer, and HIV/AIDS) is projected to be subject to disease management by 2010 (Scott 1999; Institute for the Future 1999).

Program Development

Disease management program development involves many steps, consistent with any population health management strategy. First, as described
in Chapter 3, the perspective of the program must be identified in order
to establish the framework of the disease management strategy. Part of
defining program perspective involves the important step of agreeing upon
program goals. It is important to consider issues such as: Why is this program being developed? Is a disease management strategy being developed
as a way to improve quality and clinical outcomes? Are accreditation standards or quality improvement goals a concern? Is lowering medical expenses
a primary goal? Are there other factors such as developing relationships
with employers or improving patient satisfaction that should be considered? (McAlearney 2000).

Next in the program development process, as described in Chapter
3, a target population must be defined. Due to the significant burden of
prevalent chronic illnesses such as congestive heart failure (CHF), coronary artery disease (CAD), diabetes mellitus, and asthma, these are among
the most common targets for disease management. Targeting populations
by disease status makes many diseases potential candidates, and programs
have emerged in multiple clinical areas. In addition to these common

illness conditions such as low back pain and acquired immune deficiency syndrome (HIV/AIDS), a number of more rare and catastrophic illnesses are also good candidates for programs. This variety of targets is described in both this chapter and in Chapter 8 on catastrophic care management.

Selection of diseases for disease management should attempt to follow program goals that are being or have been established for such an initiative. Selecting chronic illnesses for disease management should follow several criteria (Plocher 1997; McAlearney 2000).

- The disease is associated with a high volume of visits to physician providers or emergency departments, hospitalizations, and is very expensive to manage based on other utilization criteria.
- There is a high percentage of preventable complications associated with the disease.
- The disease is highly prevalent within the target population.
- A disease management program can show an effect within a short time frame such as one to three years.
- The chronic condition can be managed in the outpatient setting using low technology and nonsurgical interventions.
- Treatment of the disease is associated with high rates of patient noncompliance, but the noncompliance is amenable to change through patient education.
- A high rate of variability exists among current practice patterns.
- Payers such as employers would be interested in reducing some of the indirect costs of the disease, such as absenteeism and worker productivity.
- The disease is associated with high rates of preventable utilization such as emergency department visits or hospitalizations.
- Treatment for the disease is characterized by multiple referrals to multiple providers.
- Guidelines for optimal patient treatment exist or there is the potential to develop these practice guidelines.
- Clinical consensus is achievable about how to define quality of care, which outcomes to select for measurement, and how to improve clinical outcomes for this disease.

After identifying target diseases for a program, another issue is how to manage comorbidities and whether additional disease management initiatives must be undertaken to address these associated comorbidities (e.g. heart disease and problems related to diabetes). Management of multiple conditions can add complexity to disease management programs, and providers must have an appropriate strategy to address these issues.

Next, depending on characteristics of both the disease and the population targeted, individual members of the target population must be identified. Evidence to support the success of disease management programs is growing; however, the evidence selected to justify resource investment must

FIGURE 7.2

Percent of
Care of Six
Conditions
(Diabetes,
CHF, COPD,
Asthma,
Cancer, and
HIV/AIDS)
that Will Be
Subject to
Disease
Management

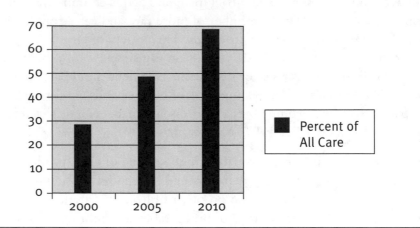

SOURCE: Institute for the Future; modified from Scott, L. 1999. "It's All in the Delivery; Disease
Management: The Right Care at the Right Time." *Modern Physician* (September) 1: 30–40.

be valid and reliable. Data sources such as medical claims, surveys, and
pharmaceutical claims may all be helpful, as well as referrals from physicians and other care providers (Chapter 4 describes this identification process
in further detail). Determining the appropriate sources of information to
properly identify individuals for a disease management strategy—and then
developing ways to encourage targeted persons to participate—is crucial.

Disease management program development should continue similar to the development process for other population health management
strategies. Activities such as data management, development of care process
tools, patient education, and evaluation are all critical. Depending on the
nature of the disease selected, the population targeted, and the processes
used to identify individuals, different program components may require
more or less attention. (Chapters 11 through 14 address some of these
additional program development issues).

Patient Issues

From a patient perspective, participating in a disease management program
offers many benefits. Disease management programs often use a patient-
centered model that puts patient needs first. Patients typically receive education about their disease and are trained in disease self-management methods. Most disease management programs also develop ways to improve
communication and coordination among healthcare providers—clearly a
benefit to patients. Programs attempt to use proven methods and can achieve
success by reducing utilization rates and improving satisfaction for patients
with chronic diseases. Furthermore, patients who keep chronic illnesses

under control reduce the incidence of complications related to their diseases, enabling them to maintain better health.

Participation in most disease management programs confers a considerable amount of responsibility on patients to comply with treatment regimens. In many ways, disease management programs are more patient management than disease management (Roughan and White 2000). Patients involved must take steps to supervise their disease progress and attempt to improve their health behaviors in areas such as medication adherence, diet, and monitoring their illness. Patients must also communicate with providers about their disease status, often on a daily basis. Patients who do not appreciate this level of constant awareness and concern may feel burdened by a disease management program that has been developed "for their own good." Instead, they may resent outside intrusion into activities and personal choices.

One of the most important components of a disease management program is education. Studies have shown that patients with chronic illnesses decrease their rates of hospital readmissions when they receive education about how to manage their diseases. Among different educational approaches, patient education videos are emerging as a popular component of many disease management programs. According to Milner Fenwick, Inc., of Baltimore, Maryland, a producer of patient education videos, over 90 percent of homes have video equipment and video ranks second only to print materials for communication distribution. Furthermore, when patients' families and friends can hear the same message about healthy behaviors and disease management that patients receive, they are more likely to be involved in helping patients to change behaviors (Egger 1999). Using educational videos helps to support the concept of a multidisciplinary disease management approach with the patient at the center.

Designing disease management programs around patient-centered outcomes is another important consideration. While clinical and cost measures may be of primary interest to program sponsors, patient outcomes such as functional status, quality of life, and personal well-being are also critical to measure. By collecting information directly from patients through questionnaires and surveys, patient-centered outcomes can be monitored and evaluated (Roughan and White 2000). Use of such data collection tools helps programs focus on information relevant to patient participants and helps caregivers tailor programs to the needs of individual patients.

Emphasizing the central role of the patient and overcoming patient resistance to participation clearly present challenges to program development. Although putting patient needs first is consistent with standard clinical practice, ensuring constant monitoring and follow-up may require a new approach. Trying to balance the patient's need for autonomy with appropriate clinical management can be a critical issue affecting program success.

Evidence

The challenge of evaluating a program both fairly and comprehensively is another critical program development issue. Some past studies highlighting program successes may have been overly optimistic because of poor study design or inappropriate research methodologies.

To assess program impact, both active participants and those patients who did not participate must be included in the evaluation. This inclusive criterion is appropriate because it is the entire population of individuals with the disease who have been targeted—not just willing participants— that is relevant to the organization that is financially and clinically responsible for their care. Programs that do a phenomenal job of improving disease outcomes for willing participants but only touch a small proportion of all eligible program candidates may have less of an overall impact than programs that tailor outreach to individuals at all stages of interest and willingness to change behaviors in the targeted disease population.

Good studies of disease management impact share a number of characteristics, as reported by Diamond (1999):

1. They create a baseline measurement for utilization including events, hospitalizations, and procedures, and describe these as rates per thousand, distinguishing between whether program participants are under 65 or 65 and over.
2. A baseline economic burden of disease is determined on a per-member-per-month basis, based on over or under 65 years of age.
3. Program effects are measured as reductions in rates per thousand from the measured baseline, adjusting for age and differences in membership.
4. They measure the economic effect of the intervention per member per month for individuals under and over 65, adjusting for age and other membership differences.

Keeping these evaluation considerations in mind during program development can help ensure that program impact can be measured and reported.

As initiatives are undertaken in conjunction with appropriate evaluation efforts, it becomes easier to justify program development and investment based on supporting evidence. However, despite multiple program successes, truly long-term measurements of outcomes do not yet exist. It is hoped that initial positive results are sustainable over the long term, but studies to demonstrate this effect have yet to be published.

Given available evidence, a strong case can now be made in favor of disease management approaches as a way to both improve quality of care for individuals and reduce medical care costs. Rather than describe multiple studies showing such trends, it is illustrative to describe individual program efforts and their results. Representative programs have been selected from the following areas: health systems, health plans, provider organizations, employers, and independent vendors.

Health System: Lovelace Health System

As the second largest healthcare provider in the state of New Mexico and a subsidiary of Cigna, Lovelace Health System assumes almost full financial risk for the medical care of 233,000 people. To manage this risk, a primary strategic initiative for the organization is its disease management program. As of 1998, Lovelace had developed 19 disease management programs, called episodes of care (EOC). These programs range from pediatric asthma to low back pain, with an emphasis on those chronic conditions suffered by its patient population.

The diabetes EOC program provides a specific example of how the Lovelace disease management effort works in practice (Friedman et al. 1998). An EOC team was formed to facilitate collaboration among all professionals participating in the diabetes program and includes an endocrinologist, a primary care physician, diabetes educators, registered dieticians, a pharmacist, a quality consultant, a case manager, an administrator, and patients. Team meetings are held twice monthly to review data, analyze ongoing programs, and plan for future program expansions and implementations.

Specific features of the diabetes EOC program include the use of practice guidelines and patient interventions, along with program components that leverage the information systems capability being developed for disease management at Lovelace. Practice guidelines are consistent with those of the American Diabetes Association and help ensure appropriate treatment of participating patients. Patient interventions include focused diabetes clinic visits, patient education efforts, reminder systems for appointments and preventive exams, and "Diabetes Days," which offer patients a physician visit, blood tests, eye exams, and education, all in one extended appointment and primary care location.

As an information systems innovation, medical profile screens have been developed by Lovelace to give providers online access to patients' treatment history. Computer terminals are installed in every provider room, allowing physicians to review multiple types of patient information including demographics, medical history, laboratory values, and radiology reports. Another information systems innovation provides reports to diabetes providers so they can compare their performance with that of their peers in the greater Lovelace Health System. In addition to providing performance measurement information against a benchmark, reports also list patients who did not receive necessary tests, examinations, or services, to ensure that patients are not lost to follow-up (Friedman et al. 1998).

Clinical and financial results of the Lovelace EOC program reportedly vary widely, with some programs demonstrating improvements in care quality with no associated financial savings. For the pediatric asthma program, for example, the 225 children enrolled experienced half as many hospitalizations as they did prior to program development, but outpatient utilization increased. Although a control group population was not identified, a pre-post study design was used to measure program impact. Results showed that asthma-related claims increased from an average of $1,120 per year to $1,165 after program initiation (Scott 1999). Ongoing evaluation of this program and, ideally, use of a control group to concurrently measure changes in utilization will help the program maintain its focus on health as well as financial outcomes for patients and providers.

Health Plan: Group Health Cooperative of Puget Sound

Another disease management program has been developed for diabetics who are members of the Group Health Cooperative of Puget Sound staff model HMO. With over 200 primary care physicians treating approximately 15,000 diabetics, the program was developed to help primary care teams deliver better population-based diabetes care to their patients.

This program was developed based on models of effective care delivery for chronically ill populations and includes the following elements (Ellrodt et al. 1997):

- an on-line, continually updated registry of diabetes patients;
- evidence-based guidelines for care such as glycemic control, retinal screening, foot care, and screening for microalbuminuria;
- guidance to support patients in self-managment of their disease;
- redesign of primary care practices to encourage group visits for diabetes patients; and
- use of a diabetes expert care team (including a diabetologist and a diabetes nurse educator) to see patients along with the primary care teams.

Group Health's program, similar to the Lovelace diabetes EOC program, uses sophisticated information systems to leverage its reach and effect. Clinical information systems are linked and provide access to administrative, pharmacy, and laboratory data. The diabetes registry focuses on information relevant to diabetes and includes linked clinical and administrative data. Diabetic patients are identified through a combination of administrative, pharmacy, laboratory and hospital discharge data, and providers are given a quarterly report that identifies diabetic patients in their practice. This summary report also provides information about dates and results of routine examinations such as lipid levels, serum creatinine levels, and retinal examinations.

The Group Health Program is widely viewed as a success with both patient and provider satisfaction levels demonstrating improvement. From a clinical process perspective, screening rates for retinal eye screenings, foot examinations, and microalbuminuria and hemoglobin A1c testing all increased, demonstrating improvement in both quality of care and patient compliance with treatment regimens (McCulloch et al. 1998).

Provider Organization: Santa Clara County IPA

Another model for disease management program development is for providers to directly offer the program. This approach makes particular sense when providers are at risk for the medical care costs of their patients because of risk contracts delegated to them through managed care organizations. Santa Clara County Independent Practice Association (IPA) is a San Mateo, California-based IPA with 800 doctors supporting 130,000 capitated HMO patients. Interested in reducing its medical care expenses, the group launched disease management programs for heart failure and asthma in 1997.

With a number of allergists in the IPA, the group chose to launch the asthma program in-house. However, for the heart failure program, the IPA worked with a vendor for the first year to develop the initial program. The 150 patients enrolled in the CHF program send daily reports to the IPA on weight, blood pressure, and other clinical measurements. This information is reviewed over a secure Internet site by nurses who follow up with patients or who alert physicians about patients who need direct contact. Program results have not been rigorously evaluated, but preliminary findings have encouraged the IPA to continue their disease management effort. A simple pre- and post-comparison shows that hospital days have fallen at least 20 percent while costs for specialty physicians have also reportedly dropped. Patient satisfaction with the program is also reportedly high, and 93 percent of patients enrolled say they understand their conditions better, while 88 percent report they feel more confident about taking care of themselves (Scott 1999).

Employer: First Chicago NBD

Programs offered through employers offer one alternative to disease management program development from the provider side. A diabetes disease management program developed in the mid-1990s by First Chicago NBD (now Bank One) proved to be very encouraging. First Chicago developed a work-site program for employees in the Chicago area and used information from medical claims and short-term disability absences to identify employees with diabetes. Under the heading of work-site education, a diabetes disease management program was developed that included educational seminars given by a diabetes health educator on topics such as nutrition and meal planning, exercise, medication, prevention of complications, and managing stress.

After only three months in the program, results were very positive. Participants' mean fasting blood glucose levels dropped 9.2 percent, mean glycosolated hemoglobin levels dropped from 11.5 percent to 10.1 percent, and mean hemoglobin A1c levels dropped from 9.0 percent to 8.3 percent. The rate of annual eye exams was 59 percent among study participants compared to the national average of 39 percent reported by the National Committee for Quality Assurance. Such promising initial results encouraged First Chicago as they anticipated fewer days absent, fewer short-term disability days and lower medical costs related to diabetes as a result of this program (Burns 1998; Burton and Connerty 1998).

Health Plan Working with Independent Vendor: Humana and Cardiac Solutions

One example of a program developed by a vendor in coordination with a health plan is a CHF disease management program that vendor Cardiac Solutions has implemented at Louisville, Kentucky-based Humana, Inc. Using the carve-out program from Cardiac Solutions, based in Buffalo Grove, IL, Humana reported a 58 percent decrease in hospital days and a 49 percent decrease in emergency department visits. Cardiac Solutions focuses on patient education and physician involvement as it attempts to alert physicians to clinical problems as early as possible. In collaboration with Humana, 4,933 patients with congestive heart failure (CHF) were enrolled in the Cardiac Solutions program. After accounting for the program's operating cost and the firm's fees, total medical expenses for patients in the program decreased by 52.6 percent, or by $33 million over two years (Scott 1999).

The Cardiac Solutions program relies on nurses as a link between patients and physicians to both help educate patients about their disease and increase medication compliance. A major focus of Cardiac Solutions' program has been on patient education and the actual process of how to best educate patients. Over time, the company reports that they learned that it was best to provide patients with one-on-one education over the telephone and break up educational topics into smaller sessions with less information per session (Scott 1999). A combination of an initial home visit from a nurse along with multiple health assessments and planned education programs delivered over the telephone have been the backbone of this vendor's approach ("Humana" 1998).

Cardiac Solutions provides disease management services for 10,000 people suffering from cardiovascular disease, chronic obstructive pulmonary disease, congestive heart failure, or diabetes. They have contracts with 30 health plans and report $40 million in annual revenues (Scott 1999).

Independent Vendor: Pfizer Health Solutions

Pfizer Health Solutions, the clinical informatics subsidiary of New York-based Pfizer Inc., developed a clinical information system called the Clinical Management System (CMS) to support disease management in a variety of settings. By integrating data from various sources, the CMS disease management programs are designed to provide proactive outpatient monitoring services that then enable early medical intervention by physicians and other providers.

Implementation of the Congestive Heart Failure (CHF) Management Program using the Clinical Management System at the New York Medical Group resulted in reductions of CHF-related expenses while patient health status and quality of care were either maintained or improved. Initial 12-month outcomes showed participating patients either maintained (95 percent) or improved (2 percent) their status on the New York Heart Association Class Designations (Class I-IV) (Pfizer Health Solutions 2000), compared to patients receiving usual care who typically maintain (46 percent) or worsen (46 percent) over time (Smith 1999). Costs associated with inpatient CHF care were reduced by 2.4 times that of the group receiving usual care, and both patient and provider satisfaction with the program were very good (Pfizer Health Solutions 2000).

Collaboration between Pfizer Health Solutions and Wellpoint Health Networks, Inc. created the successful "Love Your Heart" program for individuals with heart disease. Using the Clinical Management System, the program was implemented for approximately one-third of the eligible study population. Early results reported for 61 percent of the population at 6 months showed reductions in cholesterol of 20 points, an increase of 24 percent for individuals using diet to manage their weight, an increase in 13 percent using exercise, and a 15-percent increase in smoking cessation. Patient satisfaction levels of 100 percent were also reported, with 64 percent as very satisfied and 36 percent as satisfied (Pfizer Health Solutions 2000).

Additional work for Pfizer Health Solutions has focused on public programs. A collaborative effort in Maine with the ME-Cares project was selected by the Health Care Financing Administration as a Medicare demonstration project for its coordinated care initiative. Focused on cardiovascular disease outcomes, the project uses Pfizer's Clinical Management System software in the 17 Maine hospitals that have been participating in the project with the company Medical Care Development. The demonstration is encouraging 10 more hospitals to join the group, so that 73 percent of the hospitals in Maine (80 percent of the state population) will be participants in the study ("Report" 2001; Pfizer Health Solutions 2000).

Conclusion

Optimistic predictions about the future of disease management hold that its distinction as a different approach to healthcare provision will disappear. Instead, predicts the Institute for the Future, a think tank based in Menlo Park, California, disease management will be part of the usual care process as a model for care delivery (Scott 1999).

With the expansion of the Internet, it is expected that disease management approaches will be modified in multiple ways to make them both more accessible to patients and providers, as well as more effective. The incorporation of new technologies and new developments in information systems capabilities should make integrated disease management approaches completely consistent with medical management and patient-focused care. These opportunities and challenges are discussed further in Chapter 14, "Information Technology."

Acknowledgment

The author is extremely grateful to Ryan Minic for early background research leading to this chapter and to Emily Cruz for her research assistance with this information.

REFERENCES

Agency for Health Care Policy and Research (AHCPR). 1999. *Selected "Greatest Hits" of Outcomes Research at AHCPR.* Rockville, MD: U.S. Department of Health and Human Services.

American Diabetes Association. 2002. "Facts & Figures: The Impact of Diabetes." [On-line information; retrieved 1/31/01.] http://www.diabetes.org/ada/facts.asp.

American Heart Association. 2001. [On-line information; retrieved 1/31/01.] http://women.americanheart.org/ and http://americanheart.org/.

Barnett, P., A. W. Cohen, L. A. Emma, J. Jacobson, P. Kjerstad, M. W. Koch, N. D. Kohatsu, A. Lewis, M. Mettler, E. C. Nelson, S. Poole, C. Reisinger, P. Terry, and V. C. Villagra. 1999. "Requires Physician Authorization: California Law Poses Serious Threat to DM Programs." *Demand and Disease Management* 5 (10): 153–58.

Bodenheimer, T. 1999. "Disease Management—Promises and Pitfalls." *New England Journal of Medicine* 340 (15): 1202–05.

The Boston Consulting Group. 1995. *The Promise of Disease Management.* Boston: The Boston Consulting Group Inc.

Burns, J. 1998. "Results of This Diabetes Program Are Easy to See." *Managed Healthcare* (November): 48.

Burton, W. N., and C. M. Connerty. 1998. "Evaluation of a Worksite-based Patient Education Intervention Targeted at Employees with Diabetes Mellitus." *Journal of Occupational and Environmental Medicine* 40 (8): 702–06.

"California Law Poses Serious Threat to DM Programs." 1999. *Healthcare Demand and Disease Management* (Oct.): 153–55.

Diamond, F. 1999. "Disease Management's Motivation Factor Can Skew Study Results." *Managed Care* 8 (6): 45–46, 49–50.

Disease Management Association of America (DMAA). 2002. "Definition of Disease Management." Washington, DC: DMAA. [On-line information; retrieved 5/7/02.] http://www.dmaa.org/definition.html.

Egger, E. 1999. "Education gaining integral role in managed care's disease management efforts." *Health Care Strategic Management* 17 (3): 21.

Ellrodt, G., D. J. Cook, J. Lee, M. Cho, D. Hunt, and S. Weingarten. 1997. "Evidence-based Disease Management." *Journal of the American Medical Association* 278 (20): 1687–92.

"Employers Interested in Disease Management—If It Brings a Return." 1998. *Managed Care* (April): 44A-H. [On-line article; retrieved 2/12/02.] http://www.managedcaremag.com/archives/9804/9804.dsm_employers.pdf.

Epstein, R.S., and L. M. Sherwood. 1996. "From Outcomes Research to Disease Management: a Guide for the Perplexed." *Annals of Internal Medicine* 124 (9): 832–37.

Friedman, N. M., J. M. Gleason, and M. J. Kent. 1998. "Management of Diabetes Mellitus in Lovelace Health Systems' Episodes of Care Program." *Effective Clinical Practice* 1 (1): 5–11.

Gervitz, F., R. R. Corrato, P. Chodoff, and D. B. Nash. 1999. "Chronic Disease, Women's Health, and 'Disease Management': The Latest Trend?" *Women's Health Issues* 9 (1): 18–29.

Gillespie, G. L. 1999. *Disease Management: Balancing Cost and Quality.* Reston, VA: The National Pharmaceutical Council.

Gurnee, M. C., and R. V. DaSilva. 1997. "Constructing Disease Management Programs." *Managed Care* 6 (6): 67–70, 75–76.

"Humana CHF Program Cuts Costs, Admissions." 1998. *Healthcare Benchmarks* 5 (12): 173–75.

Institute For the Future. 2000. "Weaving Disease Management into the Fabric of Patient Care." Menlo Park, CA: Institute for the Future. [On-line information; retrieved 2/4/01.] http://www.iftf.org/html.

Joshi, M. S., and D. B. Bernard. 1999. "Classic CQI Integrated with Comprehensive Disease Management as a Model for Performance Improvement." *Joint Commission Journal on Quality Improvement* 25 (8): 383–95.

McAlearney, A. S. 2000. "Designing and Developing Effective Disease Management programmes: Key Decisions for Programme Success." *Disease Management and Health Outcomes* 7 (3): 139–48.

McCulloch, D K., M. J. Price, M. Hindmarsh, and E. H. Wagner. 1998. "A Population-based Approach to Diabetes Management in a Primary Care Setting: Early Results and Lessons Learned." *Effective Clinical Practice* 1 (1): 12–22.

Musich, S. A., W. N. Burton, and D. W. Edington. 1999. "Costs and Benefits of Prevention and Disease Management." *Disease Management and Health Outcomes* 5 (3): 153–66.

National Committee for Quality Assurance (NCQA). 2001. "NCQA Releases Final Disease Management Accreditation and Certification Standards." Washington, DC: NCQA. [On-line information; retrieved 2/21/02.] http://www.ncqa.org/Communications/News/dmfinalstds.htm.

Novartis Pharmecauticals. 1998. *Pharmacy Benefit Report: Trends and Forecasts 1998 Edition.* East Hanover, NJ: Novartis Pharmecauticals.

Partnership for Solutions. 2001. *Prevalence and Cost of Chronic Conditions.* Baltimore, MD: Partnership for Solutions. [Online article or information; retrieved 2/6/02.] http://www.chronicnet.org/statistics/issue_briefs.htm; http://www.chronicnet.org/statistics/prevalence.htm.

Pfizer Health Solutions. 2000. [On-line article; retrieved 2/13/02.] http://www.pfizerhealthsolutions.com/main.htm; http://www.pfizer-heatlhsolutions.com/pr_052501.htm; and http://www.pfizer.com/pfizerinc/about/press/jackson.html

Plocher, D. W. 1997. "Disease Management." In *Essentials of Managed Health Care,* 2nd Ed., edited by P. R. Kongstvedt. Gaithersberg, MD: Aspen Publishers, Inc.

Pomerantz, J. M. 2000. "Behavioral Health Matters: Will Behavioral Carveout Management Companies Shift to Disease Management?" *Drug Benefit Trends* 12 (2): 2–8.

"Prevention and Disease Management Are Worth the Investment." 1999. *Drug & Therapeutic Perspectives* 14 (12): 14–16.

Rabinowitz, E. 2001. "Disease Management in Medicaid Plans: Moving Health Care into the Patient's World." *Healthplan* 42 (6): 20–24.

"Report on Medicare Compliance." 2001 (March 15). [On-line information; retrieved 3/15/01.] http://www.aishealth.com/GovernmentNews.html#anchor243015

Ritterband, D. R. 2000. "Disease Management: Old Wine in New Bottles?" *Journal of Healthcare Management* 45 (4): 255–66.

Roughan, J., and E. B. White. 2000. "Making Disease Management Patient-centric." *Health Management Technology* 21 (6): 46–48.

Scott, L. 1999. "It's All in the Delivery; Disease Management: The Right Care at the Right Time." *Modern Physician* (September) 1: 30–40.

Todd, W. E., and D. Nash. 1997. *Disease Management: A Systems Approach to Improving Patient Outcomes.* Chicago: American Hospital Publishing, Inc.

"Two Managed Medicaid Plans Lead Way in Serving Children with Special Needs." 2001. *Managed Medicare and Medicaid* (7/23/01); {On-line article; retrieved 1/22/02.] http://www.aishealth.com/ManagedCare/MgdCareAdvisor /TwoManaged.html.

"Two Medicaid DM Programs Point to Improved Outcomes and Cost Savings." 2001. *Managed Medicare and Medicaid* August 20. [On-line article; retrieved 1/22/02.] www.aishealth.com/ManagedCare/MgdCareAdviosr/TwoMedicaid.html.

CATASTROPHIC CARE MANAGEMENT

Catastrophic care management is a special type of disease management that focuses on catastrophic injuries and rare illnesses. In the United States, catastrophic events are estimated to account for over $30 billion in medical expenses each year. Catastrophic cases are defined as those high-severity cases that require specialized, complex management, usually involving multiple providers and multiple sites of care. However, while chronic disease management is somewhat predictable in both intensity and effect, catastrophic cases are much less common and less predictable in both occurrence and outcome. For the purposes of this chapter, rare or catastrophic conditions are those that occur infrequently enough in the population so as to be poor candidates for traditional disease management programs. Examples of conditions that are appropriate for catastrophic care management include brain injuries, severe burns, different cancers, transplants, and high-risk newborns.

Traditional candidates for disease management meet criteria such as high prevalence or specific symptoms and disease outcomes that may be modified within a short time frame. In contrast, catastrophic conditions may be associated with a high rate of variability among current practice patterns, treatment may be characterized by multiple referrals to multiple providers, and outcomes may take a longer period of time to achieve. For catastrophic injuries, a catastrophic care management strategy is similarly appropriate. Motor vehicle accidents, falls, and exposures are major contributors to the approximately 8,000 accidents per year that result in catastrophic injury (Lipold 1998). However, such injuries are not predictable with respect to their occurrence, and management of their outcomes can be improved by a coordinated care management approach.

Research has shown that a small percentage of total cases drive a large proportion of total healthcare costs. A statistic commonly used to describe catastrophic cases is that they represent less than 1 percent of all claims filed, but can be responsible for 20 to 30 percent of a payer's total costs (see Figure 8.1). Franklin Health reports that the 1998 average cost per case for those cases in Group 1 with the least severe conditions is $1,200, compared to $6,600 per case for those in Group 2 with controlled but chronic needs. In contrast, Group 3 claimants with complex care needs have average costs per case of $71,600. Proportionately, the expensive cases where complex care was needed represented less than 5 percent of total claimants compared to the lower severity cases who represented over 85 percent of total claimants ("DM Carve-outs" 1998). Managing these high-cost cases can generate substantial savings for the companies and providers involved.

Catastrophic cases are excellent candidates for management because they are subject to considerable variability in both costs and outcomes. Costs for such cases are estimated to vary as much as 500 percent for the same medical event, depending on the nature of the problem and the treatment approach. For an institution, this equates to treatment costs varying several hundred thousand dollars or millions of dollars for an individual case. Outcome variability is similarly staggering with final outcomes for patients with the same diagnosis ranging from barely stable to complete reintegration into a community (Otway 2000).

According to a recent survey by Franklin Health, Inc. and People's Medical Society, catastrophic illness is a major concern among Americans. Over half of the adults in the United States are worried about developing a catastrophic illness such as cancer or heart disease, or experiencing catastrophic trauma such as a life-threatening car accident or a similar event. A large majority of these survey respondents also reported that they do not think the current U.S. health insurance system can adequately meet their needs if they do experience one of these problems. Respondents are concerned about getting insurance coverage approved for needed treatments and coordinating care among and between doctors, hospitals, and insurance companies ("Facing" 1999).

A catastrophic care management approach helps address these concerns from both the consumer and payer perspectives. For consumers, developing programs that focus on providing comprehensive care management for catastrophic illnesses and injuries helps ensure that medical care and financial concerns will both be taken into account. Rare diseases may have target populations that are too small for traditional disease management programs, making a program very expensive on a per-member-per-month cost basis for a payer. Similarly, for payers concerned about how to cover the unpredictable and high costs of such cases, specialized catastrophic care management programs provide financial options such as carve-outs and integrated care management arrangements that help them better manage both financial and clinical outcomes.

History

As described, catastrophic cases are both infrequent and unpredictable in their costs and outcomes. Managed care organizations and hospitals who do not wish to assume this unpredictable risk for their patient population often purchase some type of stop-loss insurance to reinsure them against such cases. This provider-excess insurance coverage helps to cap losses for providers, but is only helpful to a certain level. High deductibles and large

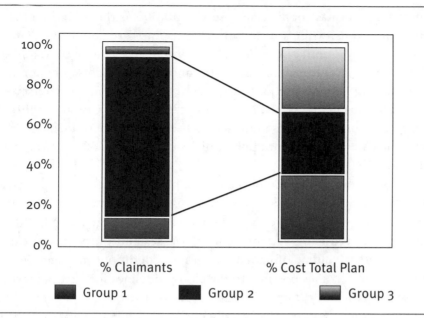

FIGURE 8.1
Health Claims
by Severity
Group

SOURCE: "DM Carve-outs Soften Sticker Shock of Catastrophic Care." 1998. *Healthcare Demand and Disease Management* 4 (6): 81–85.

coinsurance rates must still be absorbed by the risk-bearing provider organization, even in the case of provider-excess insurance coverage (Otway 2000).

Most general acute care hospitals do not experience enough of these cases to be considered experts in managing catastrophic care, and this lack of experience limits hospitals' ability to efficiently manage these cases. Specialized resources and proficiencies among the medical staff to manage such cases are difficult to develop. Furthermore, guidelines about how to best treat catastrophic cases are limited. Providers may be forced to rely on a generalized case management approach, responding to each catastrophic case as it is presented. Predictability of both outcomes and costs is incredibly difficult, and financial risk for such cases can be immense.

As a treatment alternative, many MCOs and other providers refer catastrophic cases out of their own institutions to other facilities or treatment centers that may not share the same incentive to manage costs and outcomes. However, referral institutions may not have the volume to develop appropriate guidelines for treatments, and outcome and cost variability can remain high.

One approach to identify catastrophic cases is by using claims costs. For one catastrophic care management company—Avandel Inc., of Lynnwood, Washington—cases that exceed $50,000 for treatment for a specific episode of care are considered catastrophic claims. A managed care organization—Triage Alliance, Inc., of Salem, Massachusetts—that specializes in catastrophic claims sets $100,000 as the definition for catastrophic claims, while a different catastrophic care company—Paradigm Health Corporation, of Concord, California—has a range of $150,000 to $250,000 for catastrophic cases. Still another level is used by a pharmaceutical firm—Merck & Co. Inc. in Whitehouse Station, New Jersey—that defines claims in excess of $200,000 as catastrophic (Cowans 1999). This wide range of cost figures underscores the importance of identifying catastrophic care management opportunities on the basis of more than claims cost alone.

The concept behind developing a health management approach for rare or catastrophic injuries or conditions is consistent with quality improvement techniques that strive to develop a systematic approach to health management by reducing variability in processes and outcomes of care. By increasing the volume of patients with rare conditions managed in such a program, it becomes possible to develop guidelines for best practices and more efficient healthcare utilization. Ideally, the quality of care provided for such patients can be dramatically improved while medical care costs are reduced through dedicated monitoring of the care processes and disease progression.

Many of the specialized approaches to catastrophic care management described in this chapter have developed as natural variants of disease management programs. Catastrophic care management programs have emerged primarily from two avenues: (1) from disease management companies who have developed expertise within a certain area; and (2) from insurance companies and reinsurance companies who are interested in better managing their risk for catastrophic cases. While the first catastrophic care management programs may have emerged from a special area of expertise such as cancer management, independent companies have also emerged to capitalize on this market niche. Programs that have been developed from an insurance focus tend to apply the same care management techniques to patient care processes, but may market their services to major employers more than to health plans and other providers. However, regardless of program origin, the primary reason for the existence of catastrophic care management programs is to better manage the considerable financial risk associated with such catastrophes.

Catastrophic Care Management

Catastrophic cases benefit from specialized care management for a number of reasons. First, as described above, most catastrophic cases are relatively rare, but their treatment is best managed by a great amount of specialized expertise. Patients who suffer from such conditions benefit from treatment that is multidimensional, and most catastrophic care occurs over a long period of time involving multiple facilities. Another issue is that, depending on the catastrophic event, windows of intervention may open and then close permanently if intervention does not occur. Closing of these unique windows may have lasting consequences if treatment is not initiated (Otway 2000).

Catastrophic cases are also characterized by the complexities of family and environmental considerations. When patients are unable to represent themselves, family members may be heavily involved in the treatment process. Problems may also arise from finances and insurance coverage options and limits. Environmental considerations may be relevant in cases where geographic proximity to care is an issue. Furthermore, the medical complexity of such cases makes many treatment activities longer-term in duration than acute illness management, and the involvement of multiple providers increases the need for coordination and communication to reduce both redundancies in care and variation in practice.

As described in a recent article in *Healthcare Demand and Disease Management* ("DM Carve-outs" 1998), effective management of catastrophic care cases has five common characteristics:

1. Immediate referral
2. Development of a care plan
3. Medical management by professionals with expertise in catastrophic, complex patient management
4. Individualized management
5. Patient and program satisfaction

The following discussion is adapted from this article.

Immediate Referral Process

Patients suffering from catastrophic injuries or illnesses benefit from immediate referral to a care management team. Upon identification of the catastrophic event or diagnosis of the disease, immediate referral to a team of care managers with specialized expertise in both the individual condition and the catastrophic care management process helps initiate and coordinate necessary care and support services. Catastrophic injury management programs may have referrals made within 24 hours, with care managers assigned to patients to begin the monitoring and management process. Programs that involve multidisciplinary teams may have standards in place to get teams formed and operational within two weeks of the precipitating event.

Early identification of catastrophic cases may occur through review of hospital admissions, physician referral, or referral from a hospital discharge planner. Based on the referral criteria, patients may be screened into a catastrophic care management program, a care manager be assigned, and the process be initiated by having the care manager begin meeting and communicating with involved caregivers, the patient, and the family.

Care Plan Development

Care plans are developed in a variety of ways. Catastrophic care management companies who have established databases of complex cases may be able to develop guidelines for appropriate care for different categories of cases. Most approaches involve extensive data collection that includes asking the patient and/or the family questions about clinical and psychosocial issues, home situations and family needs, relevant prior medical and psychosocial history, and other relevant issues.

Development of a care plan for an individual typically proceeds by using data collected from the case and supplementing this information with analysis of similar catastrophic cases, if such analytic capability is available. By using a comparative analysis approach, it may be possible to categorize cases by severity levels and estimate probabilities of achieving realistic outcomes from treatment.

A care plan for catastrophic care management may include a variety of components such as treatment guidelines and protocols, predictions about returning to work and productivity, resource requirements for care, and other types of analyses. Multiple people may be involved in developing the plan, including care managers, physicians, administrative staff, and analysts. The care plan must also be coordinated with the patient and/or family, especially when attempting to identify treatment preferences such as traditional or alternative medicine and aggressive or palliative care options.

Catastrophic Patient Management Expertise

Including professionals who have expertise treating and managing patients with catastrophic, complex care needs helps ensure appropriateness and efficiency in the care management process. For a catastrophic injury management program, physicians with expertise in treating severe burns, spinal cord injury, acquired brain injury, and multiple traumas expedite the care plan development process and provide a level of clinical experience to achieve the best possible outcomes with less cost and within less time.

One way to ensure availability of providers with expertise in catastrophic illnesses is to work with provider networks and centers of excellence. Contracting with vendors who have developed these relationships or who provide specialized training for their caregivers in the management of complex cases can be effective. By enlisting experts in the care of catastrophic cases, the timeframe for care management can be reduced and outcomes enhanced.

Individualized Patient Management

In catastrophic care, as in other types of care, every patient is different. While programs can provide general guidance about what to expect and what to consider for different categories of patients, recognizing that each patient is an individual case is vital. Successful catastrophic care management strategies use available data and information derived from each individual case to tailor care management interventions appropriate for the individual patients and their situations.

Patient and Program Satisfaction

Patients and family members involved in the catastrophic care management process must be satisfied with the care and services they receive. Including family members and patients in the process of planning care is very important, as is offering one-on-one education sessions and support groups as needed. By paying attention to psychosocial needs as well as clinical and financial concerns, catastrophic care management programs are most likely to be successful.

Catastrophic care management providers who have worked in this market report strong results in satisfying both patients and clients. Patients and their families appreciate being included in the care management process and knowing what potential outcomes to expect. Employers are also satisfied. Using one catastrophic care management program vendor, Paradigm, return to work for individuals with a catastrophic injury has been 35 percent, markedly better than the 10 percent average expected. Lawyers are also less likely to be involved in managed cases, as represented by a 40 to 50 percent drop in the involvement of attorneys. Similarly, health plans appreciate the savings of 10 to 15 percent in the costs of rehabilitation in the first year and 25 percent over the lifetime of the patient. Additional factors in catastrophic care management can also reduce costs by using group purchasing arrangements, coordinating durable medical equipment needs, and coordinating medication administration ("DM Carve-outs" 1998).

Managing Catastrophic Illnesses and Injuries

Management of catastrophic illnesses and injuries is clearly very complex and expensive. Catastrophic medical problems such as kidney failure, cancer, immunodeficiency disease, severe neonatal problems, or the need for organ transplants can all lend themselves to a catastrophic care management strategy. Similarly, injuries such as severe burns, head trauma, and spinal cord injuries can be equally devastating in both clinical and economic terms. The following pages present descriptions and examples of how catastrophic care management can proceed with different illnesses and injuries.

Catastrophic Illness: Cancer

While not always considered a catastrophic diagnosis, cancer represents another catastrophic care niche that can be carved out of the healthcare risk market. The annual market for cancer care in the United States alone is estimated to be $120 billion in both direct and indirect costs.

Salick Health Care Inc. has established a network of centers across the country to provide detection, diagnosis, treatment, support, and follow-up care for individuals who have cancer and other hematological disorders. Services are marketed to payers and healthcare providers such as hospitals and physicians who may be at risk for the costs of such care. Their managed care subsidiary, SALICKNET, Inc., has specifically expanded into risk-based products for cancer care management. By applying independently derived and developed practice guidelines, SALICKNET attempts to appropriately manage risk for their clients, who include HMOs, managed care entities, self-insured employers, and other payers. The success of their approach has been demonstrated in an independent study of 100,000 members in south Florida that found 5 percent changes in reduced morbidity, decreased hospital stays, and improved quality of life for patients over nationwide averages for cancer-related care (Campbell 1996).

Vida Healthcare is another cancer disease management company and is based in Minneapolis, Minnesota. Their program emphasizes quality improvement in managing approximately 2,000 cancer patients for health plans in New England and Chicago. Clinical outcomes for the program have not yet been studied, but quality measures such as the rate of patients with Stage 1 or Stage 2 breast cancer receiving lumpectomies was reportedly 68 percent, compared to a national rate of 50 percent to 60 percent. Similarly, of a small sample of 31 patients surveyed for their perceptions of the program, 90 percent rated Vida "excellent" or "very good" (Scott 1999).

Catastrophic Illness: End-Stage Renal Disease (ESRD)

End-stage renal disease is another excellent candidate for catastrophic care management. In treating renal disease, the U.S. market for dialysis services exceeds $4 billion each year. Kidney (renal) disease is identified by the level of serum creatinine. Estimates of the incidence of kidney disease from the Third National Health and Nutrition Examination Survey (NHANES) show that 10.9 million people in the United States have elevated creatinine levels over 1.5 mg/dl, and 0.8 million have levels over 2.0 mg/dl (Jones et al. 1998). Unfortunately, end-stage renal disease (ESRD) leads to renal failure, and in 1997, nearly 80,000 persons reportedly developed ESRD. Renal failure is more common as people age, with an estimated 1,300 persons (per million) age 65 and over developing renal failure. It is also more common in Native Americans and Blacks where the rates are over four times those of white populations. Kidney failure is most commonly caused by diabetes and hypertension (67 percent of all cases), further supporting the importance of disease management strategies to address these conditions.

Given the incidence of ESRD in the over-65 population, Medicare is a major insurer covering ESRD. For 1995, 264,260 ESRD patients were served by the Medicare program, at a cost of nearly $9.3 billion. While this population represents only 5.8 percent of Medicare beneficiaries, the cost per person of $35,154 is over seven times the average cost per person for non-ESRD patients (HCFA 1997). Medicaid is believed to insure the majority of those ineligible for Medicare coverage. A study of Medicaid expenditures on ESRD in three states showed California spending $46.4 million on 1,239 ESRD patients and Georgia and Michigan each spending almost $5 million on an estimated 140 patients (HCFA 1995).

The prevalence and expense of end-stage renal disease (ESRD) in the Medicare population has made this disease an ideal target for catastrophic care management. A Medicare ESRD managed care demonstration program has been developed and is being tested in Tennessee, Florida, and California to determine the feasibility and cost-effectiveness of providing coordinated care management for ESRD patients. While the program has just been initiated, the National Kidney Foundation (2002) has expressed concern about the importance of finding providers with experience treating ESRD patients, a key factor in effective catastrophic care management. Evidence of the importance of early referral of ESRD patients to nephrologists to lower the risk of death also highlights the importance of catastrophic care management strategies to support early and appropriate referrals for the ESRD patient population ("Medicare" 1998). (See 8.1 "Renal Disease: Renal Management Strategies" at www.ache.org/pubs/mcalearney/start.cfm.)

Rare Diseases

Programs for rare diseases are especially hard to develop because the target patient population is, by definition, very small. It is not uncommon for diagnosis of rare diseases to be slow. The National Organization for Rare Disorders (NORD) of New Fairfield, Connecticut, reports that for about 35 percent of rare diseases, it takes 1 to 6 years for condition diagnosis, and for another 15 percent, it may take 7 years or more (Reynolds 1999).

The 1983 Orphan Drug Act developed a classification system for rare diseases based on the criterion that fewer than 200,000 Americans suffer from the disease. Interestingly, this standard makes all but the most prevalent cancers such as breast, lung, prostate, colorectal, and non-Hodgkins lymphoma rare diseases. Overall, 6,000 rare diseases have been identified, and the NORD maintains an online database with information about 1,100 of these disorders (Reynolds 1999).

The Internet has emerged as an information technology tool to help sufferers of rare diseases in multiple ways. One application of the Internet is to create communities among sufferers of rare diseases who may live very far away from one other. Web sites describing symptoms and potential treatments can help individuals who suffer from rare diseases. NORD attempts to bring together patients who are frustrated about limited research into their disease and spark research studies based on this shared interest. NORD also tries to match patients with appropriate clinical trials, including arranging transportation to distant trial sites by making agreements with airlines and private pilots. In a similar approach, the Association of Cancer Online Resources Inc. website (http://www.acor.org) hosts online discussion and support groups for cancer patients. Among others, these 79 groups include lists for rare cancers in general as well as specific lists for rare neoplasms (Reynolds 1999).

Another benefit of the Internet is developing a single source of medical information to help patients learn about treatment options and clinical trials. It is not only difficult for patients to find appropriate clinical trials for their diseases, but to organize clinical trials testing therapies for rare diseases (Lucey et al. 2000). NORD serves as a source of such disease-specific information, offering users reports that describe the disorders in detail. Disease-specific web sites can also provide information for both physicians and patients to improve understanding and management of rare disorders. This growing awareness helps speed diagnosis of rare diseases and also makes it possible for individuals to be referred more quickly into those catastrophic care management programs that may exist.

One catastrophic care management company, Accordant Health Services, manages 14 rare conditions including lupus and cystic fibrosis. Accordant has nine contracts that cover 7 million people including 6,000 patients with its targeted conditions. The Accordant program provides detailed descriptions of its program objectives and activities to physicians to encourage provider awareness and participation. Evaluation of Accordant's success focuses mainly on reduction of hospitalizations. Accordant reports that across all patients in their programs, hospitalizations have dropped 53 percent. A small study of 120 patients also showed a 43 percent reduction in total claims costs that was associated with a net program savings of about 20 percent (Scott 1999).

Rare Diseases: Amotrophic Lateral Sclerosis (ALS)

Catastrophic care management is very appropriate for diseases that are less common among members of the general population. Amyotrophic lateral sclerosis (ALS) is described as a chronic and incapacitating disease and is actually the most common motor neuron disease syndrome among adults. It is classified as catastrophic, as 50 percent of ALS patients die within 3 to 4 years of symptom onset and only 20 percent survive for 5 years. ALS has been defined as an appropriate target for a care management program because it offers opportunities for patient education, caregiver training, better communication among providers, and guidelines for diagnosis and treatment (Matheron et al. 1998).

A care management program focused on ALS can be developed to take advantage of disease management program components that improve the quality of patient care and increase patient satisfaction. Patients need education about both the disease and the resources available to cope with their ongoing functional losses (Matheron et al. 1998). Unfortunately, because ALS is progressive, functional losses such as speech, swallowing, and oral muscular deficits cannot be reversed, so it is important to focus on improving patient quality of life and empowering them to plan for the future.

Caregiver training is important so that physicians are better able to diagnosis ALS early and so that neurologists are aware of existing therapeutic strategies to help ameliorate symptoms and slow disease progression (Matheron et al. 1998). Communication among providers is critical, as specialists and nonspecialists work together to coordinate care for their patients. Communication with patients, families, psychologists, and other caregivers is also important to maintain focus on maximizing quality of life for affected patients. Finally, guidelines and protocols that guide the care management process can improve treatment consistency and care quality. By combining all of these components into a catastrophic care management program, the needs of both patients and families can be continually addressed in the face of a devastating and terminal diagnosis.

Catastrophic Injuries: Severe Burns and Trauma

Catastrophic injuries also lend themselves well to catastrophic care management. According to estimates developed by a catastrophic reinsurance company, the average cost of a traumatic brain injury is $500,000 and an average burn case can cost millions of dollars. Nonetheless, the frequency of these catastrophic cases is not great. As illustrated in Table 8.1, the combined frequency of 5 major catastrophic conditions is still only 49 cases per 100,000 member lives (Otway and LaPine 2000). When injuries are severe enough to cause partial or permanent disability, patients, families, employers, and healthcare providers may all be involved in the catastrophic care management process. Cases such as spinal cord injuries, severe head trauma, severe burns, and amputations may all be included.

Paradigm Health Corporation provides catastrophic injury management services and works with employers to help manage their risk. They have developed a database with information about over 2,000 catastrophic cases that are both medically complex and due to work-related injuries. Comparing individual cases with information contained in the database can help the company estimate how long an individual may need hospitalization, the types of medical procedures and care that may be necessary, the length of recovery to be expected, and prospects for that individual returning to full or partial employment (McIlvaine 1997).

The catastrophic injury management model involves careful attention to a clinical road map that includes details surrounding the injury, the risks involved in case management, and a timeline that designates how expected outcomes can be achieved. A multidisciplinary injury management team is designated for the injured worker, and both the patient and

TABLE 8.1
Frequency of
Catastrophic
Cases

Catastrophic Condition	Expected Annual Frequency (per 100,000 member lives)
Neonates	25.0
Acquired brain injury	7.0
Spinal cord injury	3.5
Multiple trauma	9.0
Severe burns	4.5
TOTAL	49.0

SOURCE: Otway, T., and P. LaPine. 2000. "Coordination Deflates the Cost of Catastrophic Cases." *Managed Care* (April): 30–31.

family become involved. This comprehensive approach to catastrophic care management helps ensure that medical, social, physiological, environmental, and family issues are all addressed (Lipold 1998).

To improve outcomes and make a positive impact for employers, Paradigm also recommends that pre-injury planning be considered. Guidelines for pre-injury planning include the following five steps (Costigan 1999):

1. Understand the problem of catastrophic injury cases and recognize that these cases differ from other lost-time claims.
2. Develop and educate a team to act in the case of catastrophic accident or injury.
3. Understand how catastrophic claims will be adjusted and meet the adjuster.
4. Evaluate the ability of your healthcare benefits provider to manage catastrophic cases.
5. Ensure that risk managers stay involved in catastrophic cases. (See 8.2 "Catastrophic Care Management: Avandel, Inc." at www.ache.org/pubs/mcalearney/start.cfm.)

Approaches to Catastrophic Care Management

A number of strategies have been developed to provide catastrophic care management services. Approaches to catastrophic care coverage include intensive case management, negotiating discounts with providers, and developing contracts with vendors that delegate all financial risk in exchange for set fees (Cowans 1999).

To provide illustrations of catastrophic care management in practice, four different strategies are described here with specific examples of their applications:

1. Centers of excellence
2. Carve-outs
3. Dedicated insurance
4. Integrated insurance and catastrophic care management

Centers of Excellence: Organ Transplants

The most prevalent application of the centers of excellence model is in the area of organ transplants. According to the United Network for Organ Sharing (U.N.O.S.) in Richmond, Virginia, more than 20,000 organ transplants were completed in U.S. hospitals in 1996. Hospitals completed tens of thousands of bone marrow and cornea transplants, which translated into substantial medical care and follow-up costs. Surgery and five years of follow-up care for organ transplants (excluding cornea) range in cost from an average of $70,300 for pancreas transplants to $364,200 for liver transplants. In combination, experts estimate that transplants cost U.S. payers more than $5 billion each year (Bell 1997).

Although many hospitals may say they can do organ transplants, there is a distinct advantage for care management programs to use facilities that specialize in such procedures. Hospitals that have experienced transplant surgeons can typically lower the risk of complications that may occur, contributing to better outcomes for patients as well as payers. Consequently, most large insurers have developed networks of preferred transplant providers and centers of excellence for transplants. These networks compete with reinsurers and case management firms who have developed their own networks of providers.

One risk of relying on a center of excellence model is that employers may be faced with different approved centers based on who is involved. Claims administrators may have different centers of excellence than those offered by utilization management firms and stop-loss insurers; therefore, it is important for the employer to resolve these conflicts so that care and coverage can be coordinated (Greenwald 1999).

The development of transplant networks has been met with favorable responses from both patients and payers. Patients have proved willing to travel outside their local areas to receive a transplant, in contrast to treatments for other conditions, which tend to be more locally based. Furthermore, approval from the Health Care Financing Administration (HCFA) for transplant centers of excellence has made Medicare reimbursement both possible and reasonable (Greenwald 1999). Employers are currently designing benefit plans to encourage employees to use centers of excellence if they are available. A typical insurance plan may provide 100 percent coverage if an employee agrees to go to a center, but only 80 percent coverage if an employee goes elsewhere. Plans may also cover travel and accommodations and a support person if employees go to recommended centers of excellence (Greenwald 1999).

Centers of Excellence: Catastrophic Care Management

As another example, Health International, based in Scottsdale, Arizona, administers catastrophic care and disease management programs for large employers using care management principles. The catastrophic care management programs rely on Health International's registered nurses who act as care managers for the program. These care managers, working with board-certified physicians, review patient treatment plans and compare them to best practices to try to improve healthcare delivery for enrollees. Disease management programs are also available to provide health information and coordinate care for diabetes, asthma, heart disease, and other chronic conditions.

Catastrophic care management services rely on centers of excellence as referral sites for enrolled patients. For patients in need of catastrophic care such as organ transplants, certain cancer treatments, or cardiac procedures, Health International refers the patient to a center of excellence. This referral is based on the patient's condition and overall health circumstances, and patients are able to choose to use the center of excellence or remain with their original provider. If a patient chooses to use the recommended center of excellence, Health International coordinates with the patient's personal physician to transfer the patient to the Center. The health plan also covers expenses for transportation, lodging, and meals for the patient and one member of the patient's family if the recommended center is not local (White 1999).

General Motors is one of the large employers using Health International to provide catastrophic care management for its employees. The total cost of healthcare for GM's 1.5 million covered lives is about $4.5 billion each year (White 1999). Use of the Health International program can save money for both the employer and employees as waste and inappropriate care are eliminated.

Another version of the centers of excellence model is used by Triage Alliance Inc., of Salem, Massachusetts. Triage Alliance negotiates discounts with healthcare providers and sends catastrophic cases to facilities that specialize in a patient's particular problem. Multiple contracts with employers, reinsurers, and stop-loss insurers have given Triage Alliance approximately 1.5 million covered lives and this volume of potential patients helps them to negotiate substantial discounts with healthcare providers. Triage Alliance believes that greater volume for healthcare facilities helps improve the chances of better clinical outcomes for patients because facilities are more prepared to deal with complex cases and handle medical complications. Payer clients reimburse Triage Alliance on a case-by-case basis (Cowans 1999).

Avandel, Inc., of Lynnwood, Washington, also uses a centers of excellence model in its development of catastrophic care networks around the United States. Rather than covering only organ and tissue transplants, Avandel's Catastrophic Care Network covers multiple events such as severe burns, traumatic injuries, catastrophic cancers (i. e., leukemia and lymphoma), and babies with severe medical conditions. The catastrophic care network includes physicians and healthcare facilities that use the best available treatment guidelines for catastrophic illnesses and injuries. In many cases, Avandel has helped to develop these guidelines by using multispecialty physician panels and information from their claims database.

Avandel's network includes 50 centers of excellence hospitals in the United States as well as 150 supporting institutions to expand the catastrophic network to most locations in the country. The Avandel Centers of Excellence include hospitals such as the Cleveland Clinic Foundation (Cleveland, Ohio), Johns Hopkins Health System (Baltimore, Maryland), Dana Farber Cancer Institute (Boston, Massachusetts), City of Hope National Medical Center (Duarte, California), Memorial Sloan Kettering (New York), and the M.D. Anderson Cancer Center (Houston, Texas). Avandel has also established a research partnership with Partners HealthCare System of Boston to focus on outcomes research including severity adjustment, treatment methodologies, and quality of care for catastrophic cases ("Avandel" 1999).

Carve-Out Model

Based in Concord, California, Paradigm Health Corporation has developed a carve-out model for catastrophic care management. Paradigm specializes in managing severe burns and trauma cases and uses an injury management team approach. After the catastrophic event, a team develops an appropriate care plan and delivers it to the covering insurance provider within two weeks. Paradigm assumes financial risk using case rates, making the program attractive to payers who prefer to transfer only the most severe risk cases. This carve-out approach allows payers to more easily predict costs for catastrophic events ("DM Carve-outs" 1998).

Rather than contract for a specific amount of treatment time, Paradigm agrees to cover all costs associated with a catastrophic claim until a defined outcome is reached. Outcomes are agreed upon based on analyses of physical, social, and emotional factors as well as all clinical issues related to the case. Paradigm's clients are able to work with Paradigm to select an appropriate outcome—ranging from hospital discharge to a patient's ability to return to work—for each case. A set fee is established that covers all services needed to achieve that defined outcome (Cowans 1999).

Paradigm's approach has apparently been successful and they have managed around 3,000 catastrophic cases out of 1.5 million covered lives. Insurance providers have been satisfied with the Paradigm model because the early intervention and early warning facilitates development of a treatment plan that typically delivers both excellent clinical outcomes and savings. Paradigm's catastrophic care management program has produced savings on these claims that average between 25 percent and 33 percent ("DM Carve-outs" 1998).

Bundling Services for Catastrophic Care Management

PharMerica, a pharmacy benefits manager based in Tampa, Florida, provides an example of offering bundled services for the purposes of catastrophic care management. This company provides medicine and durable medical equipment for patients who have catastrophic or chronic care needs. Their PharmaCare Complete service line provides a single source for home delivery of pharmaceuticals, medical supplies, medical equipment, home healthcare, and other specialized services and equipment. Patient education materials are also available, including a book listing products to help patients with activities of daily living while building strength, managing pain, and improving well-being. The service begins upon discharge of the patient from a hospital or rehabilitation facility ("DM Carve-outs" 1998). (See 8.3 "Coordinated Pharmaceutical Care" at www.ache.org/pubs/ mcalearney/start.cfm.)

Dedicated Insurance

Celtic Life Ins. Co. is an example of an insurance company attempting to develop a market for organ transplant insurance. Recognizing the major financial risk associated with organ transplants, Celtic began selling transplant policies in 1995 and by 1996 covered 70,000 lives responsible for $1.7 million in premiums. The standard Celtic insurance policy provides 100 percent reimbursement for all major organ transplants up to $2 million. Another plan provides 100 percent reimbursement up to $5 million, includes more types of bone marrow transplants, and covers 100 percent reimbursement for home healthcare services. Celtic has negotiated arrangements with 20 transplant centers throughout the United States and focuses on these centers of excellence to promote the best clinical outcomes (Bell 1997).

Integrated Insurance and Catastrophic Care Management

As with other population health management approaches, catastrophic care management programs must be developed with properly aligned incentives for both providers and payers. Medical and financial incentives are both of interest, and effective programs must take each into consideration when defining program outcomes and success. A combined approach to catastrophic care management includes provider excess insurance coverage with care management services and is offered through Keenan HealthCare of Torrance, California. This program takes into account the needs of both the patient and the at-risk entity to properly align incentives. For hospitals or managed care organizations, this strategy includes a reliable stop-loss insurance policy, but focuses catastrophic care in an outcomes-based care management approach (Otway 2000).

Similar to other strategies, this integrated approach relies on a care management team to immediately respond to catastrophic cases. Upon identification of a catastrophic case, the care management team is formed, consisting of a local nurse network manager, a medical director for the case, and clinical specialists and other catastrophic experts as needed. Ideally, these team members are selected because they have expertise and have experienced good outcomes working with a particular type of catastrophic case. Additional members of a care management team work on administration of the case and cost negotiations with providers. Together these individuals are committed to providing consistent, high-quality care that is focused on the patient and strives to attain a defined outcome (Otway 2000).

Defined outcomes for patients are established by comparing each individual patient's case-specific information to similar catastrophic cases tracked in a database. Using this data-based approach, it is possible to predict realistic outcomes and establish treatment goals for each patient. When appropriate, care pathways can be used to help the catastrophic care management program progress toward outcome goals.

The nature of a catastrophic event and other patient characteristics define expected outcome levels for patients. Because not all patients can be expected to make a full recovery, six outcome levels have been established that range from physiological instability to productive activity (Otway 2000). An integrated catastrophic care management program will typically stay in place until the expected outcome is achieved, whether this is transfer to a home setting or transition to activities within the community. Follow-up with the patient and family occurs one year after the care management program has delivered the intended outcome. By maintaining this contact and follow-up, programs can improve the accuracy of their outcome data as well as the quality of their service and patient care (Otway 2000).

Conclusion

Catastrophic care management strategies rely on specialized disease management services to focus on relatively rare and expensive cases. By helping to coordinate care and manage multidimensional treatments, catastrophic care management programs can be very successful at both reducing costs and improving outcomes. Combining patient and family education, patient self-care options, and multidisciplinary team management of catastrophic cases, clinical, financial, and psychosocial outcomes can be maximized for these patients with complex care needs.

REFERENCES

"Avandel Creates America's Largest, Most Comprehensive Catastrophic Care Network." 1999. *PR Newswire* October 8.

Bell, A. 1997. "Transplant Carveouts Slice Out a Niche." *National Underwriter*, (August 4): S-30.

Campbell, S. 1996. "Providing the Continuum of Care and Disease Management for the Catastrophically Ill." *Health Care Strategic Management* (September): 3.

Costigan, M. R. 1999. "Keying on the Worst of the Worst." *Risk & Insurance* (April 1).

Cowans, D. S. 1999. "Employers Have Various Options in Covering Catastrophic Care." *Business Insurance* (August 2).

"DM Carve-outs Soften Sticker Shock of Catastrophic Care." 1998. *Healthcare Demand and Disease Management* 4 (6): 81–85.

"Facing Serious Illness in America." 1999. *PR Newswire* (May 17).

Greenwald, J. 1999. "Employers Try to Control Catastrophic Costs." *Business Insurance* (February 1).

Health Care Financing Administration (HCFA). 1997. "Persons Served and Program Payments for Medicare Beneficiaries, by Type of High-cost User: Calendar Year 1995." *Health Care Financing Review* (Statistical Supplement): 50.

Health Care Financing Administration (HCFA). 1995. "Excluded from Universal Coverage: ESRD Patients Not Covered by Medicare." *Health Care Financing Review* 17 (2): 123.

Jones, C. A., G. M. McQuillan, J. W. Kusek, M. S. Eberhardt, W. H. Herman, J. Coresh, M. Salife, C. P. Jones, and L. Y. Agodoa. 1998. "Serum Creatinine Levels in the US Population: Third National Health and Nutrition Examination Survey." *American Journal of Kidney Disease* 32 (6): 992–9.

Lipold, A. G. 1998. "Concentration on Catastrophic Cases Helps Paradigm Cut Clients' Comp Losses." *BNA's Workers' Compensation Report* 9 (16): 411–12.

Lucey, J. F., K. S. Gautham, and A. Kappas. 2000. "Crigler-Najjar Syndrome, 1952–2000: Learning from Parents and Patients About a Very Rare Disease and Using the Internet to Recruit Patients for Studies." *Pediatrics* 205: 1152–53.

McIlvaine, A. 1997. "Data Power in Profile." *Risk & Insurance* (June).

Matheron, L., K. Barrau, and O. Blin. 1998. "Disease Management: The Example of Amyotrophic Lateral Sclerosis." *Journal of Neurology* 245 (Supp. 2): S20–S28.

"Medicare Coverage Changes Force a DM Approach to ESRD." 1998. *Healthcare Demand and Disease Management* 4 (12): 184–86.

National Kidney Foundation. 2002. "Medicare Managed Care for End Stage Renal Disease Patients." [On-line information; accessed 2/21/02.] http://www.kidney.org/general/pubpol/medicare.cfm.

Otway, T. 2000. "Managing Catastrophic Care by Aligning Clinical, Financial results." *Health Care Strategic Management* (January): 14–15.

Otway, T., and P. LaPine. 2000. "Coordination Deflates the Cost of Catastrophic Cases." *Managed Care* (April): 30–31.

Reynolds, T. 1999. "Celebrity's Death Spurs Interest in Rare Cancers." *Journal of the National Cancer Institute* 91: 2070–71.

Scott, L. 1999. "It's all in the Delivery; Disease Management: The Right Care at the Right Time." *Modern Physician* (September 1): 30–34.

White, R. 1999. "GM Tunes Up Health Plans: Managed Care Tools Help to Control Fee-for-service Costs." *Business Insurance* (March 15).

WEB SITES

PersonalPath Systems, Inc.
http://www.personalpathsystems.com, accessed 3/9/01

Franklin Health
http://www.franklinhealth.com/home.htm, accessed 2/13/02

Paradigm Health
http://www.paradigmhealth.com/index.html, accessed 2/13/02

Pharmerica
http://www.pharmerica.com/whatwedo/default.asp, accessed 2/13/02

Salick Health Care Inc.
http://www.salick.com, accessed 3/9/01

DISABILITY MANAGEMENT

Disability management refers to the population health management strategy of managing disability and health from the employer perspective. Defined as attempts to reduce the incidence of and costs associated with disability in the workplace, this topic is included in an overall discussion of population health management because of its importance in managing and maintaining the health and well-being of a specific, defined population—those who are employed. While disability management may seem less relevant to some individuals, especially to those who are not employed, the expenses of disability and associated lost time from work affect the population as a whole. Productivity in the workplace allows employers to compete effectively and maintain their market position. Furthermore, money saved on benefits costs can be used for other productive investments.

In many organizations, the disability management process is very proactive, with labor and management working together to develop and coordinate workplace-based interventions and services. Disability prevention strategies, return-to-work programs, and rehabilitation treatment options are included in a comprehensive strategy designed to reduce the personal and economic costs associated with injury and disability in the workplace (Fitzpatrick and King 2001). This chapter describes disability and the costs associated with disability, presents strategies for disability management, and concludes with a discussion of the employee perspective in disability management.

Disability Defined

Disability is defined in different ways by various entities. The Americans with Disabilities Act defines disability as "a physical or mental impairment that substantially limits one or more major life activities" (Richardson 1994; Public Health Law 1990). The National Council on Disability (1999), a federal agency that helps make recommendations to the government about issues affecting those 54 million Americans with disabilities, emphasizes that the definition of disability should be inclusive and flexible. They highlight the importance of including not only people with limiting impairments but individuals who have a history of these impairments, and persons who are perceived by others to have such impairments. A third definition of disability often used in practice states that someone is disabled if they are "limited in daily activities by their condition" (National Academy on an Aging Society 1999).

Work-Related Disability

Whether caused by injury or illness, the prevalence of disability in an employed population creates a significant opportunity for health management in the workplace. From an employer perspective, disability is a major problem. Data from the Bureau of Labor Statistics (BLS) from 1998 show that 6.7 in every 100 workers have a work-related illness or injury each year accounting for around 5.9 million injured workers. Of those 5.9 million incidents, 2.8 million were associated with lost time (BLS 1999; Fitzpatrick and King 2001).

Injuries

Considering injuries alone, a survey of industrial medicine physicians conducted by the care management organization Managed Comp Inc. found that across the United States, almost one in four occupational injuries results in lost work time of at least three days (Zolkos 1998). These delays in returning injured employees to work appear to be related to issues such as employers not allowing modified duty, employers who permitted modified duty but did not have modified duty jobs available, and treating physicians who were unwilling to force employees to return to work. Additional reported problems included the inability of the treating physician to determine work restrictions and limitations, disparities between accounts of the injury between the employee and the employer, insufficient information about the demands of the job, and conflicts of opinion among treating physicians. These findings provide support for the concepts that much of the lost time associated with workplace injuries is indeed preventable and that this issue can be addressed by an appropriate disability management strategy (Zolkos 1998).

Chronic Conditions

The prevalence of chronic conditions among workers is another common source of disability. As reported by the Robert Wood Johnson Foundation (1996), lost productivity added a cost of $234 billion to the direct cost of chronic conditions in the United States in 1990. The National Academy on an Aging Society analyzed data from the 1994 National Health Interview Survey on chronic conditions among workers and reported the following percentages of problems among workers ages 45 to 64 (not mutually exclusive):

- hearing impairments (62 percent);
- orthopedic impairments (61 percent);
- hypertension (59 percent);
- arthritis (53 percent); and
- heart disease (51 percent).

These top five chronic conditions were associated with workers experiencing a number of difficulties in the labor force. Workers with chronic conditions generally earn less money, are more frequently absent from work, and are more likely to retire from work early than their counterparts who do not have chronic conditions (National Academy on an Aging Society 1999).

Mental and Behavioral Problems

Disability due to mental and behavioral health problems is another major employer concern because of its profound effect upon worker productivity. *The Global Burden of Disease* reported that in 1990 depression was the leading cause of disability in the world, affecting nearly 51 million persons, or 13.2 percent of the world's population (Murray and Lopez 1996; Norquist and Hyman 1999). In the public sector, 26.4 percent of Social Security Disability Insurance (DI) disabled worker beneficiaries had mental disorders. In the private sector, 9.0 percent of total claims for group long-term disability insurance and 13.1 percent of the cost of all claims were reportedly due to mental disorders (Salkever et al 2000; Health Insurance Association of America 1995). Mental disorder claims for long-term disability are deemed more costly than other claims. Notably, serious mental disorders tend to affect individuals at younger ages and result in longer disability periods than other disorders. Furthermore, individuals suffering from mental disorders tend to have more difficulty returning to work than individuals with other disorders (Rupp and Scott 1995; Salkever et al. 2000). These factors all make disability due to mental illness a serious problem for employers.

Medical and Nonmedical Factors

The length of disability due to injury or illness varies widely among employees because of a combination of both medical and nonmedical factors. Medical reasons affecting the length of disability include the severity of illness or injury, access to appropriate treatment, employee age, and the course of recovery (Reed 1997; Margoshes 1998). Nonmedical factors include variation because of both psychosocial and occupational factors such as job dissatisfaction, litigation, and the relationship between an employee and the supervisor and coworkers (Margoshes 1998). These different medical and nonmedical factors are listed in Table 9.1 below.

TABLE 9.1
Reasons for
Variation in
the Length
of Disability

Medical Factors	Nonmedical Factors
• Illness or injury severity • Individual response to selected treatment • Recovery course • Stage of detection and treatment for illness or injury • Access to treatment that is effective • Medical versus surgical treatment • Age affecting time for healing and recovery, also ability to return to work (older patients take longer) • Presence of comorbid conditions, depending on nature of illness or injury • Medications, especially due to side effects (e.g., sedation)	• Psychosocial issues • Occupational factors • Relationship between work and coworkers or supervisor • Job stress • Dissatisfaction with work tasks • Policies and procedures of workplace • Prompt reporting and management of injury, accident, absence, disability • Litigation • Psychological factors including depression and anxiety • Poor information about availability of modified duty/transitional work

SOURCE: Margoshes, B. 1998. "Disability Management and Occupational Health." *Occupational Medicine* 13 (4): 693–703; and Reed, P. 1997. *The Medical Disability Advisor: Workplace Guidelines for Disability Duration*, 3rd ed. Boulder, CO: Reed Groups Ltd.

The Cost of Disability

Recent statistics provide support for the importance of considering disability in the context of an opportunity for population health management. Individuals are nine times as likely to become disabled as to die, yet most people spend little time considering disability or disability insurance. Employers, on the other hand, are very concerned about the price of disability. Census Bureau calculations predicted that disability costs would exceed $340 billion by 2000, double their level in 1990 (Hellwig 1999). A DuPont study reported that the average cost to a company associated with one missed day of work from a job-related illness or injury was $13,000. This amount includes the costs of both salary and insurance expenses, in addition to indirect costs associated with lost productivity and wages paid to replacement workers (Matthes 1992).

In 1996, the cost of accidents and injuries in the workplace exceeded $80 billion in the United States. Furthermore, employers have been estimated to spend, on average, 10 percent of payroll on those direct and indirect costs that result from employee disability (Johnson and Strosahl 1998; Fitzpatrick and King 2001). A recent research report compiled by the

Liberty Mutual Group, a leading U.S. provider of workers' compensation insurance, products, and services, calculated the proportion of workers' compensation direct costs paid for various injuries and accidents. Using data about workplace accident frequency from the U.S. Department of Labor's Bureau of Labor Statistics, their own data about workers' compensation costs, and national benefits costs estimates from the National Academy of Social insurance, they developed the picture of workplace disability illustrated in Table 9.2.

As shown in Table 9.2, the top ten injuries and accidents account for approximately 86 percent of direct workers' compensation costs, or over $34 billion. When indirect costs of workers' compensation claims are included, the total economic burden of these workplace injuries and illnesses increases dramatically, to between $125 billion and $155 billion (Liberty Mutual Group 2001). Given these staggering figures, it is no surprise that most employers are interested in disability management strategies for their defined employee populations.

From an employer perspective, the true cost of poor health and disability includes the costs associated with lost productivity. Lost productivity is measured as the costs associated with staffing necessary to replace employees who are absent from work due to short-term disability. A recent study by the Integrated Benefits Institute (IBI) reports that for a company experiencing an annual average of 20 percent absence because of short-term disability claims, the cost associated with adding workers to compensate for those absent approached $1 billion. Because those payments made to support extra workers could have been used on other capital needs for the employer, these costs were considered to represent lost productivity. Breaking down the expenses associated with employee absence, the IBI reports that only 6 percent of this cost was associated with the payment of short-term disability benefits and 18 percent was due to group health costs, while 76 percent of that expense was due to lost productivity (IBI 2001).

Medical care costs associated with disability are also an important consideration for employers. In a study of disability conducted by the IBI and MEDSTAT, medical treatments over time and associated disability payments were linked to medical episode costs to reflect the total medical and disability case cost and duration. The employer, a large manufacturing firm with 72,000 employees, reported paying $292 million for both medical and short-term disability (STD) benefits during the 2.5-year study period.

Notably, while only around 1 in 10 cases studied involved STD payments, more than half of these total medical and disability costs were accounted for by the 11 percent of cases that involved STD payments (IBI 2001). One reason for this disproportionate cost structure is that STD cases tend to involve more serious injuries, incurring higher medical and disability costs.

TABLE 9.2
Top Ten
Injuries
Resulting in
Missing Five
Days of Work
or More, 1999

Rank	Accident Causes	Percent of Workers' Compensation Direct Cost Paid, 1998	Estimated Worker's Compensation Direct Cost Nationwide
1	Overexertion (injuries caused by excessive lifting, pushing, pulling, holding, carrying, or throwing of an object)	25.5%	$10.3 billion
2	Falls on same level	11.5%	$4.6 billion
3	Bodily reaction (injuries resulting from bending, climbing, loss of balance, and slipping without falling)	9.4%	$3.8 billion
4	Falls to lower level	9.2%	$3.7 billion
5	Being struck by an object (e.g., tool falling from worker above)	8.5%	$3.4 billion
6	Repetitive motion	6.7%	$2.7 billion
7	Highway accidents	5.9%	$2.4 billion
8	Being struck against an object (e.g., a carpenter walking into a door frame)	4.3%	$1.7 billion
9	Becoming caught in or compressed by equipment	4.1%	$1.6 billion
10	Contact with temperature extremes that result in injuries (e.g., heat exhaustion, frostbite, burns)	1.0%	$0.4 billion
	Total from Top 10	86.1%	$34.6 billion
	ALL ACCIDENT CAUSES	100.0%	$40.1 billion

SOURCE: Adapted from: Liberty Mutual Group. 2001. "2002 Workplace Safety Study Released." Boston: Liberty Mutual Group. [On-line article; retrieved 7/24/02.] http://www.libertymutual.com/omapps/ContentServer?pagename=corp/Page/PressRelease

The IBI report showed that nine broad medical conditions were associated with 75 percent of the total medical and disability costs. Musculoskeletal conditions topped the list and represented 20 percent of the employer's total costs, including 40 percent of disability costs. Cardiovascular conditions were second, accounting for $39.3 million in medical and disability costs, and mental health conditions were responsible for almost $32 million in total costs, including the second largest proportion of disability costs at 26 percent (IBI 2001).

Disability Management Programs

Disability management programs are designed to reduce both the incidence and impact of disability among workers. Successful programs combine elements such as early intervention, case management, transitional work programs, and ergonomics to provide a comprehensive and proactive strategy to manage disability. Margoshes (1998) has developed a list of basic principles for disability management:

- Prevent exacerbation and aggravation
- Focus on functional ability rather than pain
- Set realistic recovery and return-to-work expectations
- Specify limitations and abilities
- Assess medical and psychosocial factors
- Communicate effectively with the patient and employer
- Consider vocational rehabilitation when indicated
- Practice recurrence management

Evidence supporting the benefits of disability management programs is strong. Programs are associated with savings to employers reflected in both lower workers' compensation costs and lower costs for disability benefits (Shrey 2000; Gice and Tompkins 1989; Bernacki and Tsai 1996). Improvements in productivity are another valued benefit for employers, especially when concretely measured by reductions in absenteeism and overall time lost from work (Shrey 1998, 2000; Carruthers 2000). Disability management programs have also been associated with favorable results such as higher employee morale, improvements in employee health and wellness, and a greater ability for employers to recruit and retain qualified employees (Carruthers 2000). Multiple studies that demonstrate positive findings as a result of instituting disability management programs (Shrey 1998) provide excellent support for this population management strategy.

The following sections describes different component parts of disability management strategies. Each of these programmatic approaches is explained, and supporting evidence is provided for their potential inclusion as part of a disability management strategy.

Prevention

Prevention is an important component of disability management because of its role in attempting to avoid injuries, illnesses, and disabilities as much as possible. From the standpoint of accident and injury prevention, programs that train employees how to perform their job functions appropriately (e.g., how to lift without injuring the back) are common in many job sites. Focusing safety programs on problematic areas (such as those shown earlier in Table 9.2) that have the most potential to negatively impact both employees and employers is crucial. Such programs can reduce employee pain and suffering, help reduce and avoid the direct costs attributable to workplace injuries, and can prevent the indirect costs of these injuries such as lowered employee morale, lost productivity, and worker replacement costs (Liberty Mutual Group 2001). As an example, an injury prevention program developed at Xerox Corp. called the Zero-Injury Strategy produced a 20-percent drop in recordable incidents for the company during the program's first year and a drop of 12 percent across all business units for the first half of 1999 (Kochaniec 1999).

Illness prevention in the context of disability management is also very important. By providing lifestyle, demand, and disease management programs in the workplace (such as those described in Chapters 5, 6, and 7), employers can ensure that these population health management strategies reach the defined and targeted employee population. Prevention measures that result in savings associated with avoidance of disease, or treatments of disease, can broadly affect the workplace when individual productivity losses do not occur because diseases are prevented. Programs such as smoking cessation, exercise enhancement, weight control, nutrition awareness, and stress management may all help prevent heart disease and can be offered in the context of an employer-focused disability management program ("Prevention" 1999). For example, one work-site program at a manufacturing company that focused specifically on controlling blood pressure estimated a benefit-to-cost ratio of 1.89 to 2.72 (Foote and Erfurt 1991). Additional evidence supporting the effectiveness of worksite prevention programs can be found in Chapter 5 in the discussion of employer-based lifestyle management strategies.

Early Intervention

Early intervention refers to programs designed to provide interventions as quickly as possible after a disabling injury or illness has occurred. Drawing from research that claims that workers actually prefer to participate productively in the workplace rather than remain absent from work and on disability (Andrews 1981), early intervention programs try to help workers continue to see themselves as valued employees of the organization. Return-to-work goals are set as soon as possible, and rehabilitation services are provided on a timely and flexible basis to accommodate the needs of the injured or ill employee. This rapid response is consistent with research suggesting that delaying rehabilitation may reduce its effectiveness (Galvin 1985).

Early intervention and early return-to-work programs have proved to be cost-effective. Research demonstrates that an important factor predicting the potential for rehabilitation success is the amount of time that passes between the occurrence of the injury and a referral to rehabilitation (Rundle 1983). Programs that incorporate immediate responses and referrals help improve return-to-work rates and lower both disability and workers' compensation costs.

General Electric Co. (GE) focused on early intervention as part of the disability management program they implemented in the mid-1980s. The program was designed to provide appropriate medical and rehabilitation services to injured or ill workers on a timely basis and coordinate such services in the best way possible. By tracking cost per worker, GE showed substantial results, including a 33-percent decrease in short-term disability, a 23-percent decrease in salary continuance and hourly sick pay, and a 35-percent decrease in workers' compensation costs (Fitzpatrick and King 2001).

Case Management

Another component of disability management programs that is also seen in other population health management strategies is case management. When dealing with workplace injuries and illnesses, case management services help ensure that disability management strategies are effectively implemented and serve as a link to plans for employees to return to work. Case management services can be provided directly through the employer, or be outsourced to vendors by either the employer or insurer.

Ideally, the case manager's role is to serve as a liaison between the employee, the employer, and other involved providers and representatives such as rehabilitation therapists, physicians, and insurance companies. Disability case managers may be trained as nurses or therapists and may have backgrounds in areas such as occupational therapy, safety management, or even workers' compensation administration.

Involvement of case managers in rehabilitation cases has been studied and the Health Insurance Association of America reports that for every dollar spent on medical rehabilitation and case management, insurers receive an average 30-to-1 return on their investment (Delvin 1996). By helping to improve communications between all involved parties, case managers can be critical partners in an effective disability management program.

Transitional Work Programs

Transitional work programs (TWPs) are typically employer-based and developed to help accommodate workers whose physical capabilities to perform regular job functions have been compromised. Such programs attempt to maintain continuing contact between employees and their employer and try to help employees return to work safely and as quickly as possible. The TWP strategy is used to integrate component job tasks that can still be safely performed, enabling employees to make a gradual transition back to work. By including program components such as conditioning, education about safe work practices, and work re-adjustment, TWPs can be a vital component of a disability management strategy (Fitzpatrick and King 2001).

One example of a successful TWP was developed by the company StorageTek, which created a transitional duty department (Fitzpatrick and King 2001). This disability management strategy helped to reduce the firm's overall lost-time costs. The program was designed to work with employees who had temporary medical restrictions that could not be accommodated in their original departments. Instead, these employees were formally transferred into the transitional duty department for up to six months, where they participated in temporary work assignments and received their full salary from transitional work. Creation of this department at StorageTek reduced days off of work from an average of 33 days per injury to 11 days per injury after three years of the program. Furthermore, the associated average lost-time indemnity cost incurred for workers' compensation claims fell from $5,000 to $1,000 with the implementation of the transitional work program (Fitzpatrick and King 2001). (See 9.1 "Transitional Work Program at Walt Disney World" at www.ache.org/pubs/mcalearney/start.cfm.)

Another successful program, the Workers Transition Network in Lancaster, Pennsylvania, is organized to help employees who have been out of work for long periods of time to reenter the workforce. Working with employer clients to help these potentially permanent disability cases, referred employees can become employees of the Workers Transition Network and receive a salary for performing an interim job. Personal counselors are assigned to referred employees to assess skills and abilities as well as interests and desires. Interim jobs are selected based on the results of the employee assessment and are typically jobs with nonprofit organizations that benefit from getting free labor from motivated but disabled workers. These interim jobs help recognize the potential contributions disabled workers can make, and the Workers Transition Network helps employees find appropriate new work, including providing assistance with resumes and performing a job search (Lerner 1998). (See 9.2 "The Transitional Work Center at Steelcase, Inc." at www.ache.org/pubs/mcalearney/start.cfm.)

Ergonomics

Ergonomics, "the science of designing jobs and tools to accommodate human capabilities" (Fitzpatrick and King 2001), is another component of disability management strategies. Ergonomics principles are applied to enhance human effectiveness at performing jobs while reducing the risk of injury from such jobs. An ergonomics program begins with a comprehensive task analysis designed to identify risk factors that may be associated with job injuries. Findings from the task analysis are then used to redesign specific job tasks to minimize injury risk factors.

Applied as part of a disability management strategy, ergonomics principles can help employers make accommodations to jobs that can allow injured employees to perform parts of their former jobs and meaningful temporary transitional work. Ergonomics can also help determine the residual work capacity of permanently injured employees so that employers can make reasonable job accommodations as stipulated under the Americans with Disabilities Act (Fitzpatrick and King 2001).

One ergonomics program success story comes from Rose Health Care, the largest medical provider in Denver. In 1995, approximately 250 cumulative stress injuries were reported in administrative departments. Using industrial hygienists and safety specialists, Rose implemented an early intervention program that included evaluating work stations and observing employees at work. From their observations, specialists recommended changes in posture and work stations, included suggestions for nonwork activities, and provided reports to the workers, the employer, and the staff physician. The cases that were targeted for early intervention showed substantially decreased average costs per case—$2,959 compared to $4,652 per case that did not receive an intervention (Fernberg 1998).

Another successful ergonomics program was implemented at Silicon Graphics, where 70 percent of the company's medical costs were attributed to upper limb disorders. Using a training program, a self-directed ergonomics resource center, and an ergonomics consultant, the firm was able to reduce reportable upper limb disorders by 41 percent in one year. Reportable cumulative trauma disorders dropped by 50 percent in the following year (Fitzpatrick and King 2001). (See 9.3 "Other Ergonomics Programs" at www.ache.org/pubs/mcalearney/start.cfm.)

Employee Assistance Programs (EAPs)

By addressing issues related to employee absence, an employee assistance program (EAP) can also be a fundamental part of an employer's disability management strategy. In fact, over 70 percent of Fortune 500 companies have implemented EAPs (Advanced Workplace Solutions 2001). These programs focus on behavioral health and family issues by helping to assess and refer employees to proper assistance resources. Providing assistance with both personal and family-related issues, EAPs can be very effective at maintaining worker productivity and reducing time off from work. Specific programs designed to deal with the problems of substance abuse and mental illness can help reduce the billions of dollars spent on accidents that produce lost time, as well as the 65 percent of workplace injuries related to the use of drugs and alcohol (Prince 2000).

The U.S. government has invested substantially in EAPs, and every federal agency now has an EAP with the goal of restoring employees to full productivity. These EAPs offer free, confidential, short-term counseling to help identify employee problems, and they can make referrals to outside organizations, facilities, or programs to assist the employee when such referrals are appropriate. Typically, the employee is responsible for following through with any referrals and for making financial arrangements for treatment if it is necessary. EAP participation is voluntary, but EAPs are available to help employees with alcohol and/or drug problems who seek rehabilitation and wish to become fully productive members of their workforce. In addition to substance abuse issues, EAPs can help address such issues as work-family balance, mental and emotional problems, family responsibilities, financial or legal difficulties, and dependent and elder care. The federal government also supports the role of EAPs in preventing and intervening in incidents involving workplace violence, delivering critical incident stress debriefings, and helping employees when agencies are restructured.

In practice, EAPs can effectively address a number of employment and disability-related issues. According to Advanced Workplace Solutions (2001), Firestone Tire and Rubber's EAP realized savings of $1.7 million, or $2,350 per person involved, while United Airlines reported a $16.35 return for every dollar invested in their EAP. General evidence about the effectiveness of EAPs shows that savings can be realized when programs are successful at identifying addictive and mental health problems early (McClellan 1990). EAPs have demonstrated recovery rates as high as 60 to 80 percent and savings on sick pay that can be dramatic (Brooks 1987). McDonnell-Douglas reports that use of their EAP was associated with reductions of 44 percent in missed work days, 81 percent in attrition rates, and $7,300 in healthcare claims filed by those who utilized the EAP. Similarly, General Motors credits their EAP with cost decreases of 40 percent in lost time, 50 percent in grievances, and 50 percent in on-the-job accidents (Advanced Workplace Solutions 2001). By focusing on prevention strategies, EAPs have demonstrated value in helping employees reduce alcohol and drug use, and in helping employers with the introduction of programs in workplace education, skills development, and changes to both policy and the work environment (Blum and Roman 1995).

On-Site Rehabilitation Clinics

Developing a rehabilitation clinic at the work site provides another opportunity to better manage workplace injuries and illnesses. The proximity of an on-site clinic to the workers treated allows rehabilitation therapists to become familiar with the activities required in actual jobs, which better enables them to assist injured workers return to work (Prince 2000). Including on-site therapists within an employer-based program of disability management also provides opportunities for injury prevention programs and other work-site wellness activities tailored specifically to employee needs.

One formal pilot study that experimented with an onsite rehabilitation center at an automobile plant found that the number of lost work days due to injury dropped from 170 in three months to only 17 in five months. Estimated savings associated with this program were $30,000, while the cost of the program was fairly small because the on-site center was not elaborate (Prince 2000).

Absence Management

Absence management programs address the fact that lost time to an employer is expensive, no matter what the reason is for the absence. Such a strategy requires combined administration or tracking of absences from numerous sources such as health, workers' compensation, long-term disability, short-term disability, the Family and Medical Leave Act, as well as vacation and personal time. Employee absence is on the rise for most employers, and a survey by CCH Inc., Chicago, reported that absenteeism cost an average of $505 per employee in 1994 ("Curbing" 1995). A recent study by the Integrated Benefits Institute showed that reasons for employee absence are typically mixed. Excluding vacation and earned time off, 37 percent of worker absences are for short-term disability, 26 percent are for incidental absence, 21 percent come under the Family and Medical Leave Act, and 16 percent are associated with workers' compensation (IBI 2000; Lipold 2000).

One example of a successful absence management program is that developed at Nationwide, a $2.8 billion company of 30,000 employees based in Columbus, Ohio. This program uses a toll-free number as the access point into an automated system that tracks and manages all employee absences. Nationwide found that after two years with this integrated absence management program, the average length of employee absence decreased by 14 percent (Lipold 2000).

Comprehensive Strategies

Disability management programs can use all or some elements of this list of program options in their attempt to better manage the health of their employee population. Comprehensive strategies have also been very successful. Three examples of these comprehensive strategies are found at Navistar International Corporation, The Long Island Railroad, and Tillsonburg District Memorial Hospital.

Navistar International, with 15,000 employees in 40 worldwide locations, used a fairly comprehensive disability management strategy to address its lost-time cases and workers' compensation costs. With aggressive safety and ergonomics programs and a closely coordinated case management program, Navistar reduced incident frequency along with decreasing lost-time cases and costs. The ergonomics program alone was associated with savings in workers' compensation costs two-thirds, from over $500,000 in 1991 to approximately $176,000 in 1997 (U.S. Department of Labor 2000).

Another comprehensive strategy was implemented by the Long Island Railroad, which combined a transitional work program, health and wellness programs, and early intervention strategies in their disability management program. After four years with this program, only 8 of the 7,000 employees reported more than one year of lost-time, in contrast to 244 workers reporting such long-term absences the prior year. This combined strategy was associated with annual savings of more than $6 million (Hursch and Shrey 1999).

As a third example, Tillsonburg District Memorial Hospital developed an effective comprehensive disability management program as their response to concerns about how absenteeism was threatening to increase medical care costs and negatively affect the quality of care delivered. This small community hospital located in southern Ontario, Canada, developed the Partners in Health program to address health and disability issues for its staff. By combining resources across the organization including those of occupational health and safety, employee health, educational services, and human resources, the Partners in Health program addressed their absenteeism problem from a multidisciplinary team approach. Program specifics included a variety of disability management strategies such as prevention, benefits management, modified work duty, case management, EAPs, and ergonomics. The program is credited with increasing awareness about the importance of attendance, improving work accommodation and/or injury or illness rehabilitation, and reducing costs associated with health and lost-time claims for the organization. This program received the 1995 Health Care Quality Team Award sponsored by the Canadian College of Health Service Executives and 3M (Caulfield 1996).

Integrated Disability Management

The concept of integrated disability management recognizes that many benefits accrue from combining the management functions for different disability and health programs under one umbrella. Traditionally, disability benefits programs have been offered and managed as distinct products, with workers' compensation separate from short-term disability, and both separate from long-term disability. The disability management framework is complicated further by completely separating administration and management of these disability-related benefits from medical or health (group health) benefits. Although benefits management for all products and programs may be administered through a common human resources department, it is common for programs to be managed as individual silos with crossover of neither personnel nor data.

Integrated disability management programs have emerged to better manage disability and medical benefits costs, which continue to increase. Because lost worker days affect employers in a similar fashion, regardless of the cause of employee absence, integrated benefits plans are especially focused on lowering absenteeism while improving worker productivity and performance. Additional benefits from an integrated program may also include improvements in employee productivity and higher customer satisfaction (Hellwig 1999), presumably because of the timely and appropriate attention paid to injured and ill employees.

One approach to integrated disability management is to use the same insurance carrier for both workers' compensation and medical benefits or for both short-term and long-term disability. Most experts, however, believe that similar results can be obtained by having different insurance plans work together toward common goals. Developing consensus and corporate policies around employer goals for reduced absenteeism and returning workers to their jobs helps align program objectives to achieve these goals.

With consensus around disability management goals, different versions of integrated disability programs can emerge. Common characteristics for these programs include a common claims intake such as a toll-free number used to submit both occupational and non-occupational disability claims; cross-trained managers in claims, workers' compensation, and disability; nurse case managers; consistent application of return-to-work protocols regardless of origin of the injury or illness; and integrated claims trend analysis that enables outcomes reporting and can provide comprehensive information about the integrated programs (Kelley 1999).

A natural starting point for integrating disability programs is to evaluate all of the organization's policies towards absences—both sicknesses and accidents or injuries—and to determine if these absences are managed. Some employers grant all requests for leave automatically while others require calls to either live or automated systems to process absences. Additional areas to consider include discipline policies, disability plans, medical plans, administration of the Family and Medical Leave Act, and any employee assistance program. Assessing all of these programs with an eye towards reducing employee injuries and illnesses as well as time lost from work enables an organization to better manage total disability costs.

The allure of integrated disability management programs for the employer is cost savings. Savings of 15 to 18 percent have been reported after employers convert to integrated programs, with some achieving cost reductions as high as 29 percent. Nonfinancial benefits—including administrative efficiencies gained and consistency with common return-to-work guidelines—can also be substantial. Well-designed plans also reduce benefits cost-shifting among programs (Storrer 2000).

Pitney Bowes Inc., a $4.4 billion mail and message management services company based in Stamford, Connecticut, developed an integrated benefits program with the goal of having healthier employees. Initially, in 1994, the company integrated group health, workers' compensation, short-term disability, and long-term disability benefits. Later the company added their wellness, employee assistance, safety, and FMLA programs to the integrated benefits whole. The integrated program also provides case management services to manage both medical treatment and return to work. Case managers assist employees interested in using the FMLA program by working with families to get family members timely and appropriate treatment and enable the employee to return to work as quickly as possible. Another opportunity for case managers is smooth referrals into the EAP to assist employees with both physical and mental health issues. Integration of benefits at Pitney Bowes has reportedly saved a considerable amount for the company in both disability claims, which have dropped 15 percent, and in the number of days lost to disability, which have decreased by 42 percent (Lipold 2000). (See 9.4 "Integrated Disability at Steelcase" at www.ache.org/pubs/mcalearney/start.cfm.)

As might be expected, available vendors can provide a wide range of disability management services. While most large employers tend to build their own integrated disability management programs, the Integrated Benefits Institute reported that as of February 2000, approximately 100 vendors were offering services ranging from consulting to integrated insurance. Standards for these vendors are still being developed, but metrics upon which to evaluate program success include employee satisfaction, the cost of benefits per employee, the number of claims filed per 100 employees, the number of lost work days per employee, and the number of injured employees per 1000 claimants who return to full work duty (Lipold 2000).

The Employee Perspective

Considering the perspective of the injured or ill employee is critical for any disability management strategy. Reportedly, only 2 percent of claimants are described as actually out to beat the system, and focusing on the 1 to 3 percent of cases involving fraud is not an effective disability management strategy (Lerner 1998). Instead, considering the needs and desires of injured or ill employees helps maintain the important connection between workers and their workplace.

Judy Lerner, a former benefits consultant who was disabled following a severe accident and chronic illness, writes about the "Ten Commandments of Good Disability Management" listed in Figure 9.1. Keeping these concepts in mind can ensure that a disability management strategy can maintain focus on the needs and circumstances of employees as well as cost-saving goals for employers.

Conclusion

Disability management programs have shown marked success in many applications. From manufacturing to service companies, disability management strategies have been able to both reduce the occurrence and cost of workplace injuries. More importantly, an effective disability management strategy can maintain employee morale and productivity which, in turn, helps to improve outcomes for both employees and employers.

1.	Make return to work a clear focus.
2.	Provide strong incentives—and no penalties—for attempting some type of work.
3.	Use the rules as guidelines, but be creative in making the most of the benefits available.
4.	Put understanding, compassionate people in positions involving contact with claimants.
5.	Establish clear and ongoing communication between claimants and the workplace.
6.	Set clear expectations of who, what, when, where, why, and how things will happen.
7.	Pay attention to the actual details of the plan in any denials and provide proper support and documentation, taking pains to comply with ERISA.
8.	Do not operate from the point of view that claimants are abusers and malingerers until proven otherwise.
9.	Avoid the abuses, excuses, delays, and deceit tactics for which some disability carriers are known.
10.	Understand that disability is a very human problem.

FIGURE 9.1

The Ten Commandments of Good Disability Management

SOURCE: Lerner, J.R. 1998. "The New Direction in Disability Management." *Business and Health* (October): 36–45.

REFERENCES

Advanced Workplace Solutions. 2001. "Proven Savings." Coral Springs, Florida: Advanced Workplace Solutions. [On-line information; retrieved 2/18/02.] http://www.employee-assistance-programs.com/Proven.htm.

Andrews, H. B. 1981. "Holistic Approach to Rehabilitation." *Journal of Rehabilitation* (April/June): 28–31.

Bernacki, E. J. and S. P. Tsai. 1996. "Managed Care for Workers' Compensation: Three Years Experience in an 'Employee Choice' State." *Journal of Occupational and Environmental Medicine* 38 (11): 1091–97.

Blum, T. C. and P. M. Roman. 1995. *Cost-Effectiveness and Preventive Implications of Employee Assistance Programs*. Rockville, MD: U.S. Department of Health and Human Services, Center for Substance Abuse Prevention.

Brooks, B. 1987. "How Alcoholic Employees Can Get Help." *Indiana Medicine* 80 (11):1102–04.

Bureau of Labor Statistics (BLS). 1999. *Survey of Occupational Illnesses: 1998*. Washington, DC: U.S. Department of Labor, Bureau of Labor Statistics.

Carruthers, M. 2000. "Disability Management Employer Coalition." *Rehab*

Management (Dec/Jan): 12, 14.

Caulfield, C. 1996. "Partners in Health: a Case Study of a Comprehensive Disability Management Program." *Healthcare Management FORUM* 9 (2): 36–43.

"Curbing Absenteeism." 1995. *HR Focus* (December): 9.

Delvin P. 1996. "Insurance Carriers Discover that Rehabilitation Case Management Generates Substantial Savings." *Work Injury Management* (May): 3.

Fernberg, P. 1998. "Health Returns from Ergonomics." *Occupational Hazards* (October). [On-line information; retrieved 5/25/01.] http://www.osha-slc.gov/SLTC/ergonomics/ergonomicreports_pub/ ergonomicsuccess/ colorado/hc001098.html.

Fitzpatrick, M. A., and P. M. King. 2001. "Disability Management Pays Off." *American Society of Safety Engineers/Professional Safety* (January): 39–41.

Foote, A., and J. C. Erfurt. 1991. "The Benefit-to-cost Ratio of Worksite Blood-pressure Control Programs." *Journal of American Medicine* 265 (10): 1283–86

Galvin, D. 1985. "Employer-based Disability Management and Rehabilitation Programs." In *Annual Review of Rehabilitation*, Vol. 5, edited by E. L. Pan et al. New York: Springer.

Gice, J., and K. Tompkins. 1989. "Return to Work Program in a Hospital Setting." *Journal of Business Psychology* 4 (2): 237–43.

Health Insurance Association of America. 1995. *Disability Claims for Mental and Nervous Disorders*. Washington, DC: Health Insurance Association of America.

Hellwig, V. 1999. "Integrating Disability Management to Help Improve the Bottom Line." *Compensation and Benefits Management* (Winter): 43–50.

Hursch, N. C., and D. E. Shrey. 1999. "Workplace Disability Management: International Trends and Perspectives." *Journal of Occupational Rehabilitation* (September): 45–59.

Integrated Benefits Institute. 2001. "Considering a New Employer Healthcare Strategy: Linking Medical Care to Productivity." *Research on Emerging Health and Productivity Issues* (February). San Francisco: Integrated Benefits Institute.

Integrated Benefits Institute. 2000. *The Integrated Benefits Institute Report on Health and Productivity Benefits* (June). San Francisco: Integrated Benefits Institute.

Johnson, P., and K. Strosahl. 1998. "The new direction in disability management: tactical teamwork." *Business and Health* (December): 21–24.

Kelley, B. V. 1999. "Health and Savings: Integrated Disability Management." *Risk Management* (November): 23–25.

Kochaniec, J. W. 1999. "Injury Prevention Efforts Targeting Behavior: Building a Safety Culture Complements Traditional Hazard Identification." *Business Insurance* (October 18): 3, 16, 20.

Lerner, J. R. 1998. "The New Direction in Disability Management." *Business and Health* (October): 36–45.

Liberty Mutual Group. 2001. "2002 Workplace Safety Study Released." Boston, MA: Liberty Mutual Group. [On-line article; retrieved 7/24/02.] http://www.libertymutual.com/omapps/ContentServer?pagename=corp /Page/PressRelease

Lipold, A. G. 2000. "Managing the Guy Who Isn't There." *Business and Health* 19 (10): 25–26; 29–30.

Margoshes, B. 1998. "Disability Management and Occupational Health." *Occupational Medicine* 13 (4): 693–703.

Matthes, K. 1992. "Companies Have the Ability to Manage Disability." *HRx and Healthcare* (April): 3.

McClellan, K. 1990. "Early Intervention into Addictive and Mental Health Disorders." *Employee Assistance Quarterly* 5 (4): 71–82.

Murray, C. J. L., and A. D. Lopez, A. D. 1996. *The Global Burden of Disease.* Cambridge, Massachusetts: Harvard University Press.

National Academy on an Aging Society. 1999. "Chronic Conditions: A Challenge for the 21st Century." Washington, DC: National Academy on an Aging Society. [On-line article; retrieved 2/18/02.] http://www. agingsociety.org/.

National Council on Disability. 1999. "Toward an Inclusive Definition of Disability." Washington, DC: NCD. [On-line article; retrieved 2/18/02.] http://www.ncd.gov/newsroom/news/f99-271.html

Norquist, G., and S. E. Hyman. 1999. "Advances in Understanding and Treating Mental Illness: Implications for Policy." *Health Affairs* 18 (5): 32–47.

Prince, M. 2000. "New Disability Management Ideas Promoted." *Business Insurance* (April): 10–11.

Public Health Law. 1990. *Americans with Disabilities Act of 1990.* [On-line information; retrieved 2/18/02.] http://www.usdoj.gov/crt/ada/ statute.html.

"Prevention and Disease Management are Worth the Investment." 1999. *Drug & Therapeutic Perspectives* 14 (12): 14–16.

Reed, P. 1997. *The Medical Disability Advisor: Workplace Guidelines for Disability Duration*, 3rd ed. Boulder, CO: Reed Groups Ltd.

Richardson, M. 1994. "The Impact of the Americans with Disabilities Act on Employment Opportunity for People with Disabilities." *Annual Reviews of Public Health* 15: 91–105.

Robert Wood Johnson Foundation. 1996. *Chronic Care in America: A 21st Century Challenge.* Princeton, NJ: Robert Wood Johnson Foundation.

Rundle, R. L. 1983. "Move Fast if You Want to Rehabilitate Workers." *Business Insurance* (May): 10–12.

Rupp, K., and S. G. Scott. 1995. "Trends in the Characteristics of DI and SSI Awardees and Duration of Program Participation." *Social Security Bulletin* 59 (1): 3–21.

Salkever D. S., H. Goldman, M. Purushothaman, and J. Shinogle. 2000. "Disability Management, Employee Health and Fringe Benefits, and Long-term-disability Claims for Mental Disorders: An Empirical Exploration." *The Milbank Quarterly* 78 (1): 79–113.

Shrey, D. E. 1998. "Effective Worksite-based Disability Management

Programs." In *Concepts and Practices of Occupational Rehabilitation*, edited by P. M. King. New York: Plenum Press.

Shrey, D. E. 2000. "Worksite Disability Management Model for Effective Return-to-work Planning." *Occupational Medicine* 15 (4): 789–801.

Storrer, S. 2000. "An Integrated Disability Management Shopping List." *Risk Management* (Nov/Dec): 56–60.

U.S. Department of Labor (OSHA). 1999. "Navistar Company Commits to Reducing Ergonomic Risks." Washington, DC: U.S. Department of Labor. [On-line article; retrieved 5/25/01]. http://www.osha-slc.gov/SLTC/ergonomics/navistar.html.

Zolkos, R. 1998. "Return-to-work Underutilized: Key to Lost Time: Survey." *Business Insurance* (April): 2.

WEB SITES

Disability Management
http://www.wbgh.org/disabilitymanagement/index.html

United States Office of Personnel Management
http://www.opm.gov/ehs/Eappage.htm

INTEGRATING POPULATION HEALTH MANAGEMENT

INTEGRATING POPULATION HEALTH MANAGEMENT CONCEPTS AND STRATEGIES

While each of the strategies presented for population health management offers opportunities for health improvement, the potential for improvement is maximized when different population health management strategies are integrated. Integration both across strategies and across different parts of the healthcare system can help improve both individual and population health outcomes.

The term *integrated population health management* reflects the different component concepts that need to be included in an optimal approach to population health management. Starting with the last term, *management*, use of this word acknowledges the important management processes that must occur on multiple levels. Individuals must manage their own health and well-being because they are in charge of their health behaviors and make choices about whether or not to seek medical care. Healthcare institutions and payers also must use management processes as they provide and pay for medical care services in single or multiple locations. Finally, physicians are involved in a clinical management process as they see patients, identify problems, make diagnoses, prescribe treatment plans, and attempt to appropriately manage diseases and treatments for the benefit of their patients.

The concept of *population health* is also multidimensional. In the context of population health management, both the health and care needs of a defined population must be managed. When individual members of a population are doing well managing their own health, staying healthy, and making appropriate decisions to seek medical care, this process is defined as self-care or self-management. However, when a self-care approach is insufficient to address illness or injury, it is important that these individuals move to the next level of care for some type of intervention. Having different population health management strategies available to address the health and care needs of the population is very important. Including physicians and other healthcare providers in this process involves contact with the healthcare system so patients can receive medical care and services. Consultations with nurses or physicians, appointments, or hospital admissions are obvious types of care that can be provided to address population

_____

See 10.1 "A Model for Population Health Management" at www.ache.org/pubs/mcalearney/start.cfm.

health problems. Ideally, patients who have accessed the healthcare system for needed advice, medications, or medical care can return to a self-care mode when their medical conditions and symptoms are in control. Patients with chronic conditions, however, or those who are temporarily or permanently disabled, maintain frequent contact with the healthcare system and may remain under the care and management of a physician or other clinician for ongoing attention and medical care. The five population health management strategies that have been discussed in this book provide a range of health and care management options that address needs of differently defined populations, from different program perspectives.

Combining the terms *population health* and *management* reflects the opportunity to help individuals manage their diseases and conditions under the guidance of appropriate providers. The notion of *integration* strengthens the individual population health management strategies by combining goals and options for health and care management. In describing the importance of integration in population health management, two types of integration are critical: (1) integration of different activities within various population health management strategies; and (2) integration of care and services across the continuum of care. With respect to the first type of integration, the formal processes of healthcare management can occur in many settings and with different targets, as seen in the preceding five chapters. By integrating different population health management strategies, from demand management to disease management to disability management, care for an entire defined population can be overseen and resources allocated more effectively and efficiently. Integration of different strategies realizes the goals of true population health management by reducing waste, improving efficiency, and maintaining focus on both health and financial outcomes.

Also important in the concept of integration is integrating health and care management across the care continuum. Formally defined, the healthcare continuum includes "a comprehensive array of health, mental health, and social services spanning all levels of intensity of care" (Evashwick and Weiss 1987). When sick individuals access the U.S. healthcare system at different places in this care continuum, fragmentation is obvious (Shortell et al. 1996). Especially when a defined population has multiple problems or when target individuals have multiple diseases, care and service provision can be very chaotic. Providing integrated population health management services helps to organize care and services from multiple providers, reimbursed by different payers, and delivered in various settings. Rather than rely upon the individual levels of the healthcare system (such as providers, payers, and the government) to coordinate their efforts to deliver and finance care, an integrated population health management strategy can optimize care and resource consumption at all levels. Care coordination is an "integrating mechanism within the continuum of care that provides the optimum in appropriate, effective, and cost-efficient care" (Evashwick and

Weiss 1987). The importance of coordination and the role of integration in population health management are discussed further in the next section.

Integration

As defined by *Merriam-Webster's Collegiate Dictionary* (1999), to integrate is "to form, coordinate, or blend into a functioning or unified whole; unite." In population health management, the process of integration helps to coordinate different health and care management activities, unifying such actions for the benefit of both the individual patient and the various components of the healthcare system. This notion of integration is also consistent with the concept of developing a sense of *systemness* in population health management (Shortell 1988; Shortell et al. 1990). Systemness reflects the ideal that each unit or division within a system comprehends its role and strategic value within the overall organization or system (Shortell et al. 1996), and integration helps to produce this unified and complete focus. By integrating population health management strategies, care and service provision are ideally coordinated to reduce errors, avoid unnecessary cost and waste, and improve health.

Shortell et al. (1996) promote the importance of integration in their work with organized delivery systems, noting that an organized delivery system is an organizational network established to provide or arrange to provide services to a defined population using a coordinated continuum of care. To function appropriately, the organized delivery system must be held accountable both clinically and financially for the health outcomes and health status of the defined population that is served (Shortell et al. 1993). Similar to the organized delivery system model presented by Shortell and others, delivery of integrated population health management strategies relies upon the ability to develop a system of care through virtual integration using contracts and strategic alliances (Goldsmith 1994; Shortell et al. 1996). While organized delivery systems are created to provide a wide range of acute and subacute healthcare services, an integrated population health management strategy focuses more on health and medical care services available beyond acute hospital care. From lifestyle management to disability management services, population health management strategies exist to promote better health and wellness in multiple settings.

In practice, it is unlikely that all components of a population health management program will be owned or controlled by a single organization. Instead, one organization or an external vendor may provide oversight, as services are delivered by different physicians and healthcare organizations and payments are made by employers, patients, and various insurers.

Gillies et al. (1993) define three important types of integration in healthcare organizations: functional integration, physician-system integration, and clinical integration. *Functional integration* refers to the integration of functional processes such as financial management, human resources, management information systems, strategic planning, marketing, and continuous quality improvement/total quality management (CQI/TQM). This functional integration may permit a system to achieve economies of scale and scope as functional components are coordinated and can produce the sense of systemness described above. Furthermore, the vision, culture, strategy, and leadership of the organization will all be positively associated with the highest level of functional integration possible. *Physician-system integration* reflects the extent to which individual physicians are linked to the healthcare organization or system economically, as well as how much they use the organization's services and facilities and participate in planning, management, and governance of the organization or system. Finally, *clinical integration* is described as the level of coordination of patient care services across caregivers, functions, activities, processes, and operational units. Ideally, clinical integration requires both horizontal integration of activities at the same stage of care delivery and vertical integration of services at different stages (Shortell et al. 1996; Conrad and Dowling 1990; Fox 1989).

From an integrated population health management perspective, these three types of integration have similar importance, with slight modifications. Integrated population health management strategies definitely benefit from functional integration, especially in the integration of information systems, communications, and CQI/TQM processes. However, because integrated population health management strategies rely upon virtual coordination of entities to deliver care and services, it is unlikely that financial or human resources efforts will be truly integrated. Instead, this strategy benefits from alignment of financial incentives, a strong emphasis on the coordination of different functional processes, and an overall perspective that recognizes the needs and values of the individual patients or participants in the program.

Next, in the context of population health management, *physician-system integration* might be better termed *provider-system integration* to reflect the wide range of physician and nonphysician providers involved in patient care and participant activities. Integrated population health management strategies may rely upon physician and care manager providers who are employed by a central population health management entity or vendor rather than by the component organizations of the virtual healthcare system. The coordination of these providers' activities with other clinical and management activities is therefore crucial.

Clinical integration is, in fact, probably the best descriptor of many of the activities of integrated population health management. Patient care services must be coordinated across multiple caregivers, functions, actions, processes, and units, as described above, regardless of stage of care delivery. Development of organizational functions such as information systems, communications processes, and CQI/TQM activities that support clinical integration can help achieve the outcome goals of better health and medical care.

These different types of integration each have strong links to the vision of integration necessary for integrated population health management. Whether integration of individual population health management strategies or integration of services across the continuum of care, optimal population health management is provided when it is coordinated and integrated. The next section describes some examples of integrated population health management in practice.

Integrated Population Health Management in Practice

An integrated population health management strategy built on functional, provider-system, and clinical integration is difficult to develop in practice. A model of how integration can promote better population health management for a target population of diabetics is illustrated in Figure 10.1, but other practical examples are emerging as well. A private managed care organization (MCO) program in Minnesota and a public-private initiative in California both demonstrate how the concepts of integrated population health management can be applied.

Minneapolis-based HealthPartners established a program called Partners for Better Health to improve the health of MCO members. Describing their process as a Population Health Cycle, they developed an improvement model based on seven steps (Isham 1997):

1. Set goals
2. Assess members' willingness to participate
3. Determine health status
4. Evaluate readiness to change
5. Design systematic interventions
6. Evaluate
7. Modify goals

Consistent with the component steps of other population health management strategies, this population health cycle was applied to a defined population of MCO members in the Twin Cities area. Goals included disease management (heart disease, diabetes), lifestyle management (breast cancer screening, childhood immunizations), and social issues (childhood injuries, domestic violence). Information from medical records, pharmacy data, laboratory results, claims data, and individual surveys was used to identify individuals and target them for intervention. Further population segmentation applied Prochaska et al.'s approach (as discussed in Chapter 5) to evaluating members' willingness and readiness to change health behaviors (Isham 1997).

FIGURE 10.1

Integration Facilitates Population Health Management of Diabetics

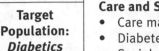

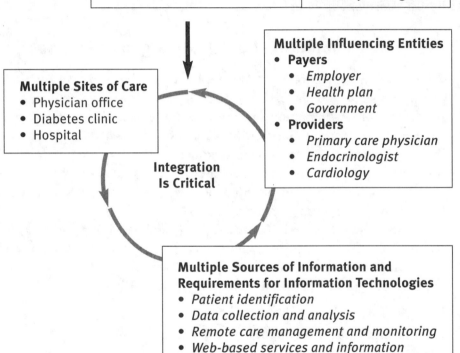

Target Population: *Diabetics*	Population Health Management Personnel Work to Coordinate Care and Services • Care manager • Diabetes health educator • Social worker • Counselor • Medical director	Program Option: *Lifestyle management*
		Program Option: *Disease Management*
		Program Option: *Disability Management*

Multiple Sites of Care
• Physician office
• Diabetes clinic
• Hospital

Integration Is Critical

Multiple Influencing Entities
• **Payers**
  • *Employer*
  • *Health plan*
  • *Government*
• **Providers**
  • *Primary care physician*
  • *Endocrinologist*
  • *Cardiology*

Multiple Sources of Information and Requirements for Information Technologies
• *Patient identification*
• *Data collection and analysis*
• *Remote care management and monitoring*
• *Web-based services and information*
• *Tracking clinical and non-clinical metrics*
• *Provider communication and coordination*

SOURCE: McAlearney, A. S. 2002. "Population Health Management in Theory and Practice." In *Advances in Health Care Management* (Volume 3), edited by G. T. Savage, J. Blair, and M. Fottler. New York: JAI Press/Elsevier Science Ltd.

Interventions for the Partners for Better Health program have been diverse. An anti-tobacco advertising campaign, called "Garbage Face," was developed for both radio and television commercials directed towards teens. Another public communications campaign strove to improve eating habits and challenged hundreds of local restaurants to create and serve low-fat and great-tasting menu items for the month of October. On the provider front, a training video was developed to teach how to recognize the symptoms of domestic violence as well as how to help members by approaching them and linking them to appropriate resources (Isham 1997). Preliminary results from the program show marked success (Isham 1997). The program goal to increase childhood immunizations from 75 to 95 percent was reached by 1997, with 96 percent of pediatric members being immunized. Breast cancer screening rates also increased, with 92 percent reporting screening, up from a rate of 86 percent in 1995. Domestic violence awareness also increased, with a 67-percent increase in the number of female members over age 40 reporting that they had been asked about safety in their personal relationships (Isham 1997).

A partnership in northern California between Stanford University, San Mateo County, and three county health plans (Blue Shield of California, Aetna, and Kaiser) provides another example of an integrated population health management strategy. The $200,000 Health Education And Risk Reduction Training (HEAR^{2}T) study program was designed "to evaluate the effectiveness of a comprehensive, individualized preventive program for people who are already at increased risk of heart disease" (Cowan 1997). With its goal of reducing the rate of hospitalizations due to heart disease by half, 350 county employees were enrolled in the program. This program integrated the concepts of disease management and lifestyle management within an overall disability management focus for San Mateo County employees. A risk assessment questionnaire was provided to employees, retirees, and their dependents, and an additional screening process stratified individuals by risk levels. Intervention options ranged from prevention activities such as risk management classes to intensive monitoring of individual cardiovascular disease risk factors. Individual counseling sessions emphasized lifestyle management issues such as smoking cessation, stress management, and improved nutrition (Cowan 1997). The HEAR^{2}T program was modeled on the successful Stanford Coronary Risk Intervention Project (SCRIP) that studied the effects of adding risk-reduction interventions to standard medical treatment. Notably, after 5 years of follow-up, the 300 SCRIP participants showed a reduction in hospitalizations of 40 percent compared to individuals with standard treatment, as well as better overall cardiac health (Haskell et al. 1994). (See 10.2 "Medicare Coordinated Care Demonstration Program" and 10.3 "Total Health Management" at www.ache.org/pubs/mcalearney/start.cfm.)

Key Components of Integrated Population Health Management

Developing an integrated population health management strategy relies on a variety of different tools and techniques, many of which are discussed in this book.

After defining the perspective and population, targeting individuals for interventions is important. However, moving beyond individual population health management strategies, an integrated population health management strategy relies upon five critical factors:

1. Aligned incentives
2. Information systems
3. Communication and coordination
4. Committed participants
5. Involved and responsive providers

Each of these factors will be discussed in the following pages. Further discussion about the tools and personnel needed to develop both individual and integrated population health strategies is presented in Chapters 11 through 14.

Aligned Incentives

One critical component of an integrated population health management strategy is that incentives be aligned to support health and wellness for participating individuals. From an employer perspective or from the perspective of society overall, it is clearly beneficial to have healthy, productive individuals—whether they are working for a company or managing their own households. Incentives for insurance companies and other payers are usually similarly aligned. By keeping individuals healthy and reducing their need for medical care services, payers benefit from having to pay less in medical care costs.

The issue of aligned incentives may become less clear if one considers the perspectives of different types of providers. Providers paid on a fee-for-service basis, whether physicians or healthcare institutions, benefit from providing service to patients. They receive reimbursement for services rendered and thus may not have any business incentive to keep patients healthy or reduce their demand for medical care. Ethically or morally they may feel some responsibility to encourage healthy behaviors among their patients, but from a business perspective, they receive less reimbursement for a population of healthy individuals that demands fewer medical care services than for a population with greater demands on the healthcare system.

Providers paid on a capitated basis or who share risk for the cost of medical care services have incentives better aligned with the goals of population health management. In such situations, these providers receive payment to cover a population of individuals (e.g., on a per-member-per-month basis) and are responsible for providing medical care to those members of the population requiring their services. Consequently, these providers have an incentive to keep their patient or member population healthy and help them make better lifestyle and self-care decisions to appropriately minimize their use of expensive medical care.

Individual patients with insurance are also at risk for the cost of their medical care because they pay for coinsurance, copayments, and any unreimbursed medical care services or prescription drugs. Quite often, individuals pay insurance premiums that correspond to their health habits (e.g., individuals who smoke have higher insurance rates than nonsmokers). This level of individual risk, however, is usually small relative to the risk burden borne by the third-party payer. While employers share the cost of health insurance premiums with their employees, employers still typically cover the bulk of the cost as an employment benefit for their employees. Other payers such as the Federal government are also responsible for the majority of medical care costs for their covered population (e.g., Medicare beneficiaries) while beneficiaries are only at risk for the cost of uncovered goods and services such as prescription drugs or long-term care. As demonstrated in the Rand Health Insurance Experiment (Newhouse 1994), making insured individuals personally responsible for a portion of the medical care services they demand makes them more likely to make appropriate decisions regarding their need for services.

Uninsured individuals typically are at risk to pay for the bulk of their medical care costs and must appeal to the benevolence of various healthcare safety net providers when they cannot pay for needed services. Interestingly, uninsured persons may have the biggest incentive to make healthy behavior choices and minimize their risks of incurring large medical care expenses. Unfortunately, however, uninsured, unemployed, and low-income persons often have difficulty with health behavior modifications because of poor access to care for preventive services. Furthermore, they are rarely members of a population targeted for health management strategies.

To create an environment of aligned incentives for an integrated population health management program, it is important that the risk of medical care costs be shared by payers, providers, and individuals. Individual patients must be sensitive to the costs of care they demand to help encourage reasonable medical care utilization decisions and increase incentives for appropriate lifestyle management decisions and healthy behavior choices. Payers must favor shared risk arrangements in which some of the risk for medical care costs is delegated to providers, some shared by individual patients (e.g., copayments and coinsurance), and the rest retained by the payer. Physician providers must share some financial risk for the care of their patients to have an incentive to encourage healthy behaviors and provide appropriate medical care. Similarly, institutional providers must be at some level of financial risk to facilitate the development of appropriate health management strategies such as disease management programs, health education strategies, and demand management strategies.

Creating a shared risk environment in the context of integrated population health management may not be easy. However, if all involved parties have some level of financial responsibility for the medical care delivered, these parties have incentives to attempt to make appropriate choices about that medical care. Having an incentive to help individuals who are members of a defined population make good choices about health and behavioral risks can promote a healthier culture overall. When no party receives financial benefit from inappropriate medical care utilization, an environment is created that encourages reasonable and appropriate allocation of healthcare resources.

An integrated population health management strategy fosters this environment. Demand management strategies can be integrated with disease management programs whenever appropriate, regardless of the source of the program. Catastrophic care management programs address issues of unexpected demand for medical care due to accident or catastrophic injury as well as providing disease management services for very expensive or rare conditions. Meanwhile, disability management programs can use the most appropriate programs available to reduce injury risk and help maintain worker health and productivity.

From the perspective of involved providers, care managers focus on the spectrum of care needs for individual patients while physicians provide clinical care and program oversight whenever necessary. Information systems provide the backbone of the integrated program, helping to monitor individuals and their interactions with various parts of the healthcare system.

The integrated population health management strategy can function effectively for any defined population. As described in Chapter 3, whether the population is defined by the employer, the federal government, insurer, or provider, it is possible to apply an appropriate health management strategy. By creating an environment where incentives are aligned to keep members of that targeted population healthy and by using appropriate types of medical care, an integrated population health management strategy can help improve health and reduce inappropriate medical care expenditures for the defined population.

Information Systems Support

An optimal population health management strategy is also dependent on sophisticated information technologies to support and integrate health and care management services. As described in Chapter 14, information technologies can range from relational databases to decision support tools and algorithms to point-of-care technologies. Incorporation of more advanced information technologies may facilitate greater levels of coordination among different population health management strategies and permit true integration of care management services.

In practice, when participating individuals receive population health management services, this patient-caregiver interaction should be documented to enable the overall care management program to track both patient concerns and provider advice. Communications with patients can be documented along with medical care utilization. Ideally, prescriptions, tests, outpatient visits, hospitalizations, rehabilitation visits, and any other medical care utilization can be tracked and monitored within an information system capable of providing decision support for appropriate use of healthcare services.

For programs without the capability to facilitate electronic documentation and integration of information, participants and providers must rely more on clear communications and paper documentation at all stages of the care management process. Not having electronic capabilities may reduce the speed with which information is processed. In addition, reliance on paper-based systems may limit providers' abilities to have a complete care management history at their fingertips if the paper records are not immediately available. Such circumstances require increased efforts on the part of participating providers to seek care management information and pay attention to written guidelines and protocols that might be important in individual patients' health management.

Including sophisticated information technologies within a population health management framework facilitates the development of an integrated program. True integration is difficult to attain and maintain in the absence of information technologies that support real-time communications, care management decision support, and ongoing monitoring of patient and program activities and outcomes. Emphasizing the importance of such information technologies promotes an integrated population health management strategy that is both responsive to patient and provider needs and effective at improving individual and population health and well-being.

Communication and Coordination

Also critical to the integrated population health management model are communication and coordination. Given the wide variety of providers and individuals potentially involved in providing population health management services, it is very important to maintain clear communications among all parties. The integrated population health management strategy benefits from an organizational and information infrastructure—whether paper or electronic—that ideally supports the communication and coordination functions.

Regardless of the level of sophistication of information technologies used, integrated population health management programs are necessarily dependent on both verbal and face-to-face interactions among providers. Frequent communications between individual providers and caregivers permit information to be shared that may not be captured in any electronic format. Furthermore, when information is available electronically but an individual provider cannot gain immediate access to such information systems, it is incumbent upon that provider to obtain relevant information in any way possible.

Patient communication skills are also very important. Participating individuals and families must understand their circumstances and be able to make informed and reasonable choices about both their health behaviors and their program activities. Communications skills training for patients can help increase the effectiveness and efficiency of patient information seeking behavior, as well as improve their ability to communicate clearly about their medical conditions in their interactions with physicians and other caregivers (Cegala et al. 2000).

Most population health management strategies rely upon constant communication and coordination as part of their standard work routines. However, for an integrated population health management program to succeed, communication and coordination are additional keys to the notion of integration. Avoiding duplication of services, misunderstandings, and medical errors are only some of the goals of such an integrated approach. In the interest of both improved care quality and health outcomes, communication and coordination are vital.

Committed Participants

Another component of integrated population health management that promotes program success is the committed involvement of individual participants. Any population defined is comprised of multiple individuals, and it is these individuals who must take primary responsibility for their health and healthcare needs. Whether healthy employees or patients with chronic conditions, the needs and behaviors of these individuals create the opportunities for health and care management that a population health management strategy is designed to address.

The importance of a consumer focus in the health services sector is gaining popularity and visibility as individuals and patients take more charge of their health and medical care. Patients often seek their own healthcare information through the Internet, conversations with friends and colleagues, the media, and other available educational material. This growing tendency of individuals to become involved in their health decisions bodes well for the success of any population health management strategy.

However, much of the difficulty of implementing a population health management program is in getting individuals to participate and commit to the attitudinal and behavioral changes required by such programs. Clearly, quitting smoking or losing weight are not simple choices for most people. Instead, comprehensive programs have been developed to help these individuals make such choices and behavior changes. Many strategies draw from the field of psychology and recognize the importance of individuals' willingness and readiness to change behaviors as part of their programmatic strategy. Remaining sensitive to the difficulty of behavior change can help programs succeed in the face of challenging health and behavior problems.

Emphasizing the importance of a consumer focus on health and health improvement can be justified regardless of the perspective of the program sponsor. Healthier, safer individuals educated about health risks and committed to healthier lifestyles will typically make decisions that are less risky both with respect to illness and injury. Insurers and other payers benefit from this strategy because these individuals are less likely to incur the need for expensive medical care. Similarly, employers benefit by having healthier employees who are less likely to become ill or disabled. Even physicians and other healthcare providers benefit because their patients are likely to have fewer demands for medical care that could have been avoided given better attention to health habits and behaviors. Finally, society clearly benefits because, in this era of limited resources, allocation of resources can be more appropriate and based on unavoidable illnesses and accidents rather than avoidable health risks.

Involved and Responsive Providers

A fifth influential factor supporting an integrated population health management strategy is the involvement and responsiveness of multiple providers. Whether physicians or other care managers, the inclusion of these healthcare professionals in the design, development, and implementation of an integrated population health management program is essential.

Provider involvement in integrated population health management can occur on a number of levels. Designing clinical interventions, developing appropriate advice and paradigms for demand management, and providing direct care for patients are all obvious provider roles. Providers also offer valuable guidance about the details of program integration by helping to delineate or modify professional boundaries between programs and sites of care as needed.

Another component of provider involvement relates to the concept of patient-centered care. While programs may be designed around guidelines and protocols, it is incumbent upon individual physician providers to make decisions about their patients' medical care needs based on their knowledge of an individual patient's circumstances (Tanenbaum 1993). Maintaining this balance between program goals and individual health needs is the role of responsive providers as they provide population-based but individualized medical care services.

Ensuring the committed involvement of physicians and care managers will help realize the goals of integrated population health management by emphasizing coordination and goal alignment (discussed in further detail in Chapters 12 and 13). By working to involve providers at all levels in program development and intervention, program success is most likely to be achieved.

Conclusion

An integrated population health management strategy considers not only chronic disease but acute illnesses, injuries, and any other events that can result in individual use of the medical care system. While each of the different population health management strategies can work well in a variety of healthcare settings, a patient-focused approach to healthcare benefits from this integrated view of population health management services. By applying an integrated population health management strategy, appropriate options for health and care management can be selected to match the needs of both program sponsors and the individuals who are members of the defined populations being served.

REFERENCES

Cegala, D. J., L. McClure, T. M. Marinelli, and D. M. Post. 2000. "The Effects of Communication Skills Training on Patients' Participation During Medical Interviews." *Patient Education and Counseling* 41: 209–22.

Conrad, D. A., and W. L. Dowling. 1990. "Vertical Integration in Health Services: Theory and Managerial Implication." *Health Care Management Review* 15 (4): 9–22.

Cowan, K. 1997. "Getting to the Heart of the Matter." *Healthcare Forum Journal* (Nov/Dec): 35.

Evashwick, C., and L. Weiss. 1987. *Managing the Continuum of Care.* Gaithersberg, MD: Aspen Publishers.

Fox, W. 1989. "Vertical integration strategies more promising than diversification." *Health Care Management Review* 14 (3): 49–56.

Gillies, R. R., S. M. Shortell, D. A. Anderson, J. B. Mitchell, and K. L. Morgan. 1993. "Conceptualizing and Measuring Integration: Findings from the Health Systems Integration Study." *Hospital and Health Services Administration* 38 (4): 467–89.

Goldsmith, J. C. 1994. "The Elusive Logic of Integration." *Health Forum Journal* 37 (5): 26–31.

Haskell, W. L., E. L. Alderman, J. M. Fair, D. J. Maron, S. F. Mackey, H. R. Superko, P. T. Williams, I. M. Johnstone, M. A. Champagne, and R. M. Krauss. 1994. "Effects of Intensive Multiple Risk Factor Reduction on Coronary Atherosclerosis and Clinical Cardiac Events in Men and Women with Coronary Artery Disease. The Stanford Coronary Risk Intervention Project (SCRIP)." *Circulation* 89 (3): 975–90.

Isham, G. 1997. "Population Health and HMOs: The Partners for Better Health Experience." *Healthcare Forum Journal* 40 (6): 36–39.

McAlearney, A. S. 2002. "Population Health Management in Theory and Practice." In *Advances in Health Care Management* Vol. 3, edited by G. T. Savage, J. Blair, and M. Fottler. New York: JAI Press/Elsevier Science Ltd.

Merriam-Webster. 1999. *Merriam-Websters' Collegiate Dictionary, Tenth Edition.* Springfield, MA: Merriam-Webster, Inc.

Newhouse, J. P. 1994. *Free for All: Lessons from the Rand Health Insurance Experiment* Cambridge, MA: Harvard University Press.

Shortell, S. M., R. R. Gillies, D. A. Anderson, J. B. Mitchell, and K. L. Morgan. 1993. "Creating Organized Delivery Systems: The Barriers and Facilitators." *Hospital and Health Services Administration.* 38(4): 447–66.

Shortell, S. M., E. M. Morrison, and B. Friedman B. 1990. *Strategic Choices for America's Hospitals: Managing Change in Turbulent Times.* San Francisco: Jossey-Bass.

Shortell, S. M. 1988. "The Evolution of Hospital Systems: Unfulfilled Promises and Self-fulfilling Prophecies." *Medical Care Review* 45 (2): 177–214.

Shortell, S. M., R. R. Gillies, D. A. Anderson, K. M. Erickson, and J. B. Mitchell. 1996. *Remaking Health Care In America: Building Organized Delivery Systems* San Francisco: Jossey-Bass.

Tanenbaum, S. 1993. "What Physicians Know." *New England Journal of Medicine* 329 (17): 1268–71.

IMPLEMENTING POPULATION HEALTH MANAGEMENT STRATEGIES

STRATEGIC PROGRAM MANAGEMENT

The ability of a healthcare organization to apply population management strategies successfully depends largely on its strategic management and implementation skills. When considered in a strategic management framework, selection of a population health management strategy should be made as a result of a situational analysis that includes both the external and internal organizational environments (Ginter et l. 2002). Then, once the population health management strategy has been selected, the issues of *strategic implementation* and *strategic control* must be addressed (illustrated in Figure 11.1).

In strategic implementation, both service delivery and support activities become considerations. Financial incentives must be aligned so that incentives for population health management programs are consistent with institutional goals. Factors such as physician relations, patient satisfaction, and other organizational implications of a new program must also be addressed to maximize program success and outcomes improvement.

To ensure strategic control, including some type of quality improvement cycle is important to address the issues of setting objectives, measuring program performance, and modifying program activities or objectives as appropriate to achieve success. This chapter considers these different strategic implementation and control issues in the context of strategic program management.

Strategic Implementation

Implementation strategies to support adoption of a population health management strategy often are delineated as part of a value chain. Michael Porter's description of the value chain as it is used to create and sustain competitive advantage has many relevant elements for population health management program development (Ginter et al. 2002; Porter 1985). In particular, service delivery and support activities are especially important in program implementation.

Service Delivery Issues

Many issues related to service delivery become critical in the implementation of population health management strategies. This section discusses four such issues, as depicted in Figure 11.1:

1. Focus
2. Marketing and promotion
3. Operation logistics
4. Provider coordination

Focus   The effective implementation of population health management strategies first depends on focus. In this context, focus refers to the desired goals and outcomes a strategy is developed to achieve. Each population health management strategy can have a different focus overall or program goals may overlap, as seen in Table 11.1. As an example, a demand management strategy concentrates on a broad population of individuals who are, for the most part, fairly healthy. This strategy may be developed from the perspective of payers such as employers or insurers, or of patients or providers. Each of these groups may find the strategy appealing because of its focus on goals such as improving health and wellness, reducing costs, increasing productivity, and improving the appropriateness of patients' demand for medical care. In contrast, a disease management program is also concerned about cost reduction and improving health and wellness, but a major focus of this program is on improving clinical outcomes. If an organization is unable to address or impact clinical outcomes, a disease management strategy may be an inappropriate choice for population health management. (See 11.1 "Program Sponsors and Program Focus" at www.ache.org/pubs/mcalearney/ start.cfm.)

Focus is also important within population health management programs. First, focus enables program designers to develop interventions appropriate to the needs and situations of the individuals targeted. In fact, a benefit of developing a focused program is the ability to pay less attention to members of a population that fall outside the target group or who are less relevant to achieving program goals. For example, while the focus of a diabetes disease management program may seem obvious, the opportunity to focus on those diabetics to improve health and reduce cost is maximized by not diverting resources to individuals with other chronic conditions which might be similarly complex but differently managed. Similarly, stratifying an insured population into different risk categories may help identify opportunities for differently defined populations such as the "worried well" or "frail elderly." Individuals who fall into the worried well category could be targeted for health education campaigns and demand management strategies that would be inappropriate for individuals who are living with chronic conditions. Categorization of the frail elderly with multiple chronic conditions might trigger intensive case management when such individuals access the healthcare system to prevent exacerbations of identified health problems and manage *situational* concerns such as living conditions or social support.

The importance of within-program focus is consistent with the concept of "focused factories" as introduced by Wickham Skinner in the field

FIGURE 11.1
Framework for
Population
Health
Management

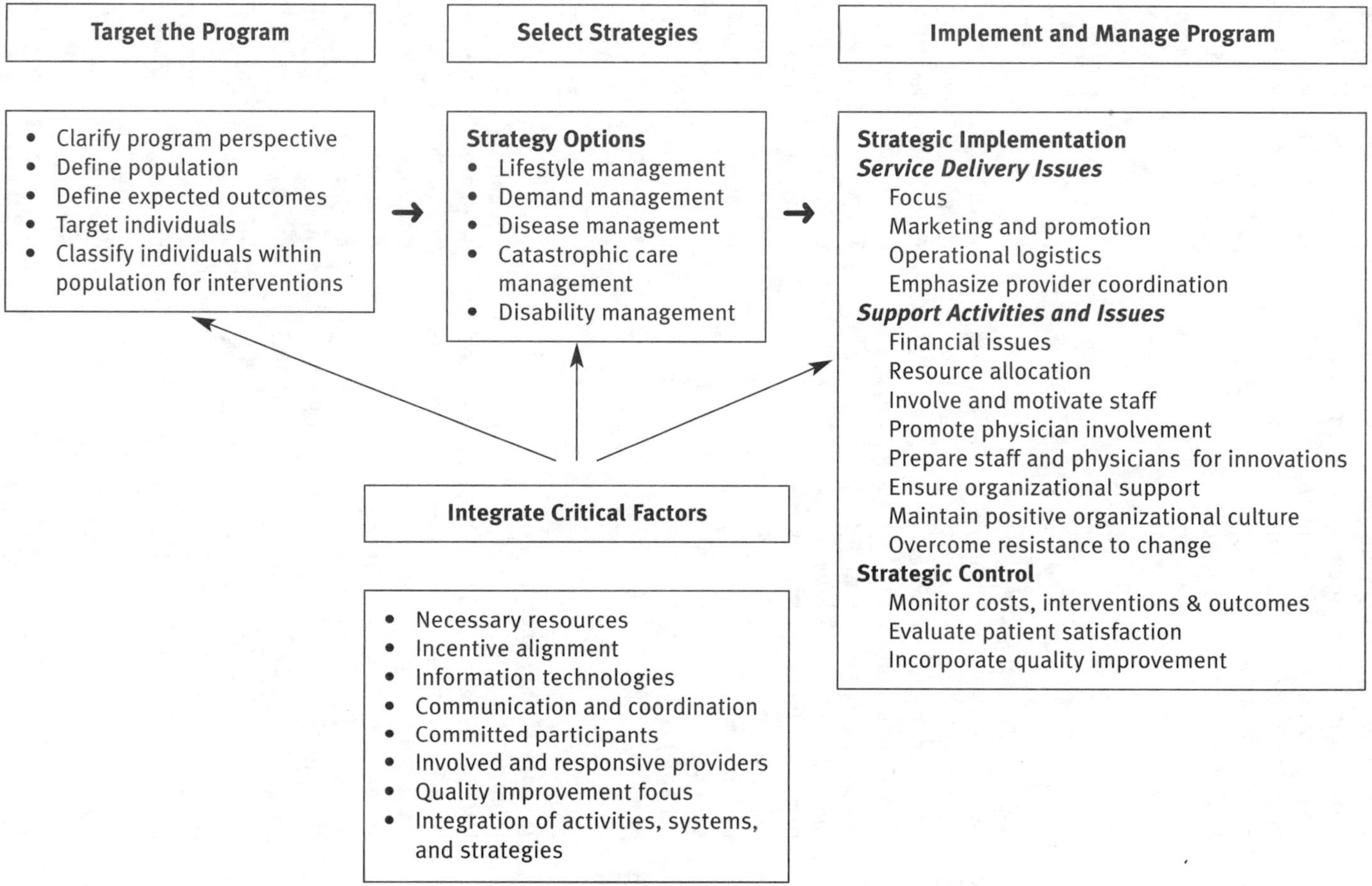

Target the Program

Implement and Manage Program

Select Strategies

Strategy Options
- Lifestyle management
- Demand management
- Disease management
- Catastrophic care management
- Disability management

Strategic Implementation
Service Delivery Issues
Focus
Marketing and promotion
Operational logistics
Emphasize provider coordination

Support Activities and Issues
Financial issues
Resource allocation
Involve and motivate staff
Promote physician involvement
Prepare staff and physicians for innovations
Ensure organizational support
Maintain positive organizational culture
Overcome resistance to change

Strategic Control
Monitor costs, interventions & outcomes
Evaluate patient satisfaction
Incorporate quality improvement

Integrate Critical Factors
- Necessary resources
- Incentive alignment
- Information technologies
- Communication and coordination
- Committed participants
- Involved and responsive providers
- Quality improvement focus
- Integration of activities, systems, and strategies

- Clarify program perspective
- Define population
- Define expected outcomes
- Target individuals
- Classify individuals within population for interventions

SOURCE: Adapted from Janet Buelow. 2002. Personal communication, February.

TABLE 11.1
Population
Health
Management
Program
Focus

Population Health Management Strategy	Relevant Perspectives	Target Population	Key Elements	Program Focus
Lifestyle Management: Help individuals make good choices about health behaviors and health risks (Chapter 5)	• Employers • Society • Government as insurer • Patients • Providers • Insurers	• Relatively healthy population groups	• Prevention strategies • Health risk reduction • Self-care focus	• Improve health and wellness • Reduce out-of-pocket cost • Improve functional outcomes • Reduce disability
Demand Management: Help individual consumers take an active role in making decisions about health and medical care needs to reduce inappropriate demand for services (Chapter 6)	• Employers • Society • Government as insurer • Patients • Providers • Insurers	• Relatively healthy population groups	• Telephone triage • Advice and referrals • Triaged counseling • Decision and behavioral support • Education to promote self-care	• Reduce cost • Improve health and wellness • Increase productivity • Improve appropriateness of demand for care • Increase provider efficiency
Disease Management: Identify individuals with certain diseases and target with specific interventions (Chapter 7)	• Society • Government as insurer • Patients • Providers • Insurers	• Individuals with chronic diseases (e.g., congestive heart failure, diabetes mellitus, asthma)	• Education, self-care information • Chronic disease monitoring and management • Clinical oversight by care managers • Coordination of care and providers	• Reduce cost • Improve health and wellness • Improve clinical outcomes • Provide appropriate care • Increase provider efficiency

TABLE 11.1
(continued)

Catastrophic Care Management:

Proactive identification of cases to provide services needed for catastrophic injuries or illnesses to improve outcomes (health and cost); may include management of medical care, rehabilitation, and end-of-life care needs (Chapter 8)	• Employers • Government as insurer • Patients • Insurers	• Individuals with catastrophic or rare illnesses, or catastrophic injuries (e.g., cancer, renal disease, injuries)	• Immediate referral to appropriate providers • Coordination of care and providers • Medical and care management by professionals with specialized expertise	• Reduce cost • Improve health and wellness • Improve clinical outcomes • Maximize functional outcomes • Reduce disability • Provide appropriate care

Disability Management:

Employer-driven initiatives to reduce lost time from work, improve worker productivity, and optimize employee health and wellness (Chapter 9)	• Employers • Society • Patients	• Employees	• Disability and injury prevention • Return-to-work programs • Coordination of care and providers • Absence management • Workplace rehabilitation	• Reduce cost • Reduce disability • Increase productivity • Reduce absenteeism • Improve health and wellness • Maximize functional outcomes

SOURCE: Adapted from McAlearney, A. S. 2002. "Population Health Management in Theory and Practice." In *Advances in Health Care Management* (Volume 3), edited by G. T. Savage, J. Blair, and M. Fottler. New York: JAI Press/Elsevier Science Ltd.

of production and operations management. As Skinner (1974) described, the notion of focused factories is based upon the idea that "simplicity and repetition breed competence." By narrowing focus on a particular service category, for instance, expertise can be developed that permits excellence and efficiency. Regina Herzlinger (1997) specifically emphasizes the importance of focus in healthcare and the opportunity for focused factories to improve both care and service, as may be realized in a focused population health management strategy.

In practice, different population health management programs can serve as versions of focused factories with different goals for their defined populations. For example, by targeting a population segment that is, in general, more healthy and able to direct their own self-care, demand management strategies use remote care management techniques to improve consumer demand, reduce cost, and improve the health and well-being of participants. Nurses can provide advice over the telephone as they apply computerized algorithms to assess callers' healthcare needs, and health education information may be delivered to all participants via the mail, outbound calls, or the Internet. This advice and educational information can be consistently offered to callers and be overseen by clinical professionals in ways to provide a standardized product, consistent with the notion of focused factories. Similarly, disease management strategies can capitalize on the concept of focus by developing clinical guidelines and protocols for the management of a particular disease and the comorbid conditions associated with it by using interventions appropriately timed and based on available evidence for their efficacy. However, in both situations, information and care can still be customized to the needs of individuals at little additional cost as providers skillfully deliver their interventions. Keeping in mind the importance of focus to develop appropriate and effective protocols and interventions can ensure program success for each population health management program.

Marketing and Promotion

The effective marketing and promotion of population health management programs among potential participants, involved organizations, and participating providers represents another critical consideration in service delivery. Even after targeting individuals for participation in such a program, getting them to actually participate may not be an easy task. Promotion and marketing of the program to individuals in certain categories of risk or health status may require that these individuals acknowledge their risky behaviors and poor health. Furthermore, for programs that rely on the willingness of individual participants to change unhealthy or risky behaviors, these individuals must be both receptive to the program and receptive to the notion of changing their behaviors. Developing appropriate messages for these potential participants can constitute a major program challenge.

Marketing and promotion throughout the organization where the program is being implemented becomes imperative. For involved providers such as physicians, nurses, and office staff, the introduction of such a program may not be a surprise. However, for other departments, gossip about new programs with goals that seem competitive or in conflict with existing initiatives often proves detrimental for employee relations. Helping organization members to see the value and recognize the perceived threat of the organizational changes inherent in new program development can be another marketing and promotion challenge.

Successful marketing and promotion tactics may differ in every organization. In a managed care organization, for example, departments such as provider relations, contracting, and even sales may be able to leverage the perceived value of implementing a population health management program. Similarly, an employer organization may be able to promote access to demand management services or lifestyle management initiatives as an added benefit for employees. Integrated disability management services may also be described favorably in communications to employees about the opportunities provided to them by their employer. In contrast, in a medical group, the opportunity to have patients with chronic diseases managed in a more holistic framework by a disease management program may be either comforting or terrifying for physicians and other caregivers, depending on existing practice patterns and models of care. Identifying potentially unfavorable reactions and developing appropriate responses for the targets of such marketing and promotional campaigns may help smooth the implementation process for both the participating organization and participants themselves.

Also, marketing population health management programs directly to physicians and other healthcare providers may be essential to ensure their participation. Program promotion may proceed as part of a general communications campaign or be part of an attempt to improve provider relations. Regardless of the approach, specifically targeting providers for marketing and promotion tactics will improve the likelihood of successful program implementation.

External marketing of new population health management programs may or may not be appropriate. Programs that attract participants with expensive medical conditions because of their reputation for good service may be valuable in improving health but create problems with financial risk (i.e., a problem of adverse selection). However, for organizations interested in promoting program benefits to employees or announcing their successes in achieving targeted health outcomes, communicating about the results of implemented programs can be very beneficial. Similarly, managed care organizations or employers may promote the availability of multiple disease management programs or of a demand management program as an added benefit for enrollees or employees within their organizations. Then, when good health outcomes are achieved, emphasizing program successes and patient satisfaction can help all involved to promote the value of carefully designed and well-implemented population health management strategies.

Operational Logistics

The logistics of program implementation create another area of management concern. Whether logistical issues focus on space needs, employee training, or detailed programmatic concerns such as incorporating a health assessment process, considering these issues early in the program design stage improves the chance of program success.

For any new program, requirements such as capital equipment or technology resources seem obvious. However, related issues must also be considered: finding space to place new equipment, creating examination room space, scheduling time for program participants, or reconfiguring work spaces to ensure privacy of telephone calls or office visits. New personnel will need appropriate equipment such as desks, computers, and so forth, but developing a dedicated population health management program such as a telephonic demand-management program may require new logistical and technology considerations not previously addressed by the organization.

Another important logistical issue is that of how employees will be introduced to a new program. Beyond the human resources issues of recruiting, hiring, training, and developing new employees, existing employees must also learn about the new program. Opportunities to work with personnel and patients involved in the health management program may be emphasized, while new requirements for documentation and communication must also be acknowledged.

When a new program leverages existing human resources, recognition of the need to accommodate new program responsibilities in addition to determining how to manage prior workload becomes crucial. Program participation may require that temporary employees be hired to backfill existing positions and free critical personnel for the new initiative. Similarly, new requirements in areas such as information systems, data management, and outcomes measurement may require consideration of additional staff to respond to new program demands.

Programs that introduce new processes may also require specific logistical attention. The example of including a health assessment process illuminates a number of potential issues. In general, health assessments can be either mailed, used on-line, or delivered telephonically. For each of these methods, however, existing organizational resources can be either helpful or can create barriers to implementation. In the case of mailed surveys, many organizations already have a process for mass mailings to enrollees, employees, or patients. Tapping into existing resources may be an obvious first step for a health management program. If existing resources are not sufficient, use of a mailing house may be an appropriate option. However, beyond the physical mailing process, logistical and managerial issues exist such as getting approvals for survey content and cover letter content, determining who will sign the cover letter or request for information, and figuring out how to obtain addresses for target respondents. Further issues may also arise such as considering the process for following up with nonrespondents, arranging a data collection process, and even establishing a "help line" for potential respondents to call with questions.

Selecting an on-line or telephonic assessment process will raise different but similarly challenging issues. On-line survey web sites will have to rely on the sponsoring institution to approve web content, security, and access. Telephonic assessments may require additional space for telephone interviewers to be housed during the survey process. And, similar to the case of mailed assessments, considerations such as telephone and electronic mail address lists, help lines, and processes for data collection and analysis must all be addressed.

Depending on the nature of a population health management program, the list of logistical issues to consider can be very long. Addressing the majority of these issues as soon as possible in program implementation becomes critically important so that such concerns become merely steps in the implementation process and not barriers to program development. (See 11.2 "Vendor and Contracting Concerns" at www.ache.org/pubs/ mcalearney/start.cfm.)

Another major service delivery issue for population health management strategy implementation is provider coordination. Providing care oversight in population health management often requires coordinating multiple provider types and locations of service to ensure quality of care and reduce duplication of activities. Primary care physicians, specialists, and hospital intensivists such as hospitalists may all be involved in the care of patients with complex conditions as they practice in their various clinics, hospitals, and outpatient offices. Care for people with chronic conditions is usually complex, increasing the possibility that medical treatments may be poorly coordinated. Population health management programs must ensure that such patients are tracked along the entire continuum of care so that they receive the services they need without duplication.

Emphasize Provider Coordination

Support Activities and Issues

Support activities are also critical in strategic program implementation. These pages describe some of the activities and issues associated with support of population health management strategies.

Financial Issues

An important goal for most population health management programs is to reduce the healthcare costs associated with the population they are serving as long as such cost reductions are not achieved at the expense of quality of care. However, depending on who holds the financial risk for the defined population targeted for health management, incentive alignment can be difficult or impossible to achieve.

As briefly described in previous chapters, the concept of financial risk in healthcare is important for a number of reasons. Financial risk associated with insurance coverage becomes relevant for potential program sponsors such as HMOs, PPOs, or other MCOs because of their insurance risk. Similarly, employers have some financial risk tied to their employees because they are financially at risk for portions of their employees' medical care coverage, as well as costs associated with employee absence and disability. Healthcare providers become concerned about financial risk if they have accepted risk from insurers. MCOs may delegate all or a portion of their financial risk to healthcare providers in the hope that these physicians and institutions will have the proper incentives to provide appropriate care and manage costs at the same time.

Organizations and provider groups reimbursed under a risk-sharing arrangement are very likely to value the potential gains of population health management programs that reduce medical care costs. These initiatives may enable MCOs and other organizations to more effectively manage their risk contracts, helping them to maintain financial viability while focusing on improved patient outcomes.

In context, in an environment where a hospital is reimbursed on a straight or discounted fee-for-service basis, hospitals are paid for the services they provide. When health management programs successfully reduce utilization and keep patients out of the hospital, the hospital may not value this program outcome because it will not provide these services. Such a reimbursement structure may make it difficult for health management programs to gain a foothold in organizations with fee-for-service reimbursement because financial incentives are not aligned. However, one opportunity for organizations considering these health management initiatives is to emphasize the importance of gains in quality of care and health status. While reimbursement goals may not be aligned, demonstrating improvements in health, patient satisfaction, and quality of care may be effective methods to improve payer loyalty or increase market share (McAlearney 2000). (See 11.3 "Carve-outs" at www.ache.org/pubs/mcalearney/start.cfm.)

Resource Allocation

The development of any population health management program requires a substantial investment of both financial and human resources. Program start-up costs for a healthcare organization may involve new employee hiring, information systems development and integration, and extensive data analyses to determine potential target persons for the program. Program development will require a substantial communications effort to share information within the organization, educate and recruit physicians for participation, and help inform payers and potential program participants about the benefits of such an initiative. These efforts must be well designed, implemented, and coordinated to ensure that health management programs have the opportunity to reach their full potential in their target population groups.

Resource allocation and financial investments can be made more predictable if programs are outsourced or carved out because many vendor businesses develop contracts that are based on fixed fees or case rates.

However, the population health management field remains a for-profit business concern for vendors, and these rates are available because such companies can effectively manage financial risk for their target populations and still retain a profit. Healthcare organizations who choose to develop programs in-house may be able to retain some of these potential program profits, but only if programs are well-designed and well-implemented. Without expertise in health management program development, it may be safer for organizations to work with outside businesses or vendors to maximize the savings potential of such programs.

Involve and Motivate Staff

The involvement and motivation of staff in any selected population health management strategy is critical. From recruitment to retention, human resource practices are important at every step in program implementation. Developing population health management programs in-house often requires hiring new personnel such as care managers or dedicated medical directors to support the new initiative. Existing staff in organizations must be retrained to perform new duties such as data collection, risk assessment, and providing telephonic interventions. The new role of care managers must be developed and supported as nurses and other clinical personnel are trained to function as comprehensive care managers. (Chapter 12 will describe these issues in more detail.)

Institutions considering adopting a population health management strategy can benefit from theory and practice in organizational development. As an example, multiple employee development opportunities exist. Nurses and social workers can receive training to become care managers, and physicians may be interested in expanding their roles to become program liaisons or medical directors. Traditional case management personnel may embrace expanded job responsibilities as care managers. Standard roles in utilization management and customer service offer opportunities to transition into new roles supporting a care management framework. Furthermore, a focus on program evaluation emphasizing the importance of measurable outcomes will introduce new opportunities in the areas of outcomes measurement, quality improvement, and health services research.

Overall, introducing a population health management approach to an organization offers benefits for employees, physicians, and patients. New job opportunities may be appealing (Hodges et al. 1998), and the opportunity for healthcare organizations to expand and fulfill their missions as providers of excellent healthcare service and outcomes can be even more appealing. Developing or reemphasizing a focus on patient-centered healthcare can invigorate clinical and administrative personnel alike. Furthermore, evidence of improved health and wellness achieved through population health management programs is attractive to both patients and providers. Leveraging the possibilities and emphasizing the opportunities inherent in a population health management focus is a key component of overall organizational strategy as a whole and can be attractive for patient, physician, and employee stakeholders as well.

Promote Physician Involvement

Another major support issue affecting the implementation of population health management programs is the integration of physicians into the process. Involvement of physician providers is not only important for patients but is critical for program success. Population health management programs that incorporate the ideas and patient care goals of physicians in the design process tend to have better experiences working with physicians to achieve population health management goals. In contrast, imposing programs on physicians without ensuring their agreement or participation often leads to difficult physician relations problems.

When physicians are not involved in a program, an inherent risk exists that care will be poorly coordinated. Not only is duplication of services a potential problem, but the risk of confusing patients by giving inconsistent clinical guidance is a real concern. Bodenheimer (1999) further argues that when commercial programs offered by independent companies are involved, the risk of poorly coordinated care may increase. If such programs select only those patients who are most motivated to change behavior, less-motivated patients and their problems are left to primary care physicians, subjecting the medical care system to further fragmentation.

One increasingly popular strategy requires physician involvement in and approval of different population health management programs. This option recognizes the importance of securing and maintaining physician participation in such programs and gives physician providers the opportunity to participate directly in program activities. Requiring physician authorization also improves program quality and professionalism because of the central role physicians will play in such authorized programs (Ritterband 2000).

Implementing a program developed with the input of involved physician providers may still be a challenge. It is highly unlikely that all physicians who will treat patient participants have been involved in program design; therefore, developing approaches to work with additional providers becomes very important. Instead of imposing population health management programs on providers, it is helpful to introduce such programs to all physicians who may be involved. Carefully planned communications campaigns can help, as will informational meetings and word-of-mouth contact between involved and uninvolved providers.

Communication efforts may be even more important in situations where an outsourced or independent program is selected for implementation. Depending on the nature of the program, some companies require physicians to participate in their patients' care management process. Disease management and catastrophic care management programs may insist that physicians use their protocols and treatment algorithms as part of program guidelines. For programs that rely less on direct physician participation such as demand management initiatives, it is still important to keep physicians well-informed about the program. Physicians seeing patients who mention that a demand management nurse recommended that they make an appointment need to know that such a referral system is in place. Overall, good quality population health management programs can enhance relations with physicians when referrals are appropriate and when patients are better and more correctly informed about their conditions than they would have been in the absence of such a program.

It is also important to keep in mind the requirements that population health management programs may impose on physicians. Programs may require additional documentation for patient care, for billing, or for treatment monitoring purposes. When programs incorporate information technology options such as automatic paging, automated reports, or other contacts with providers, they also create a different level of interaction with providers. For physicians who have not been involved in the program design process, incorporating a disease management program into their patient care routines can be very intrusive and disruptive. Dedicated communications campaigns can directly address physician and staff concerns. Additionally, inviting those providers that are interested to participate in program development and implementation often proves beneficial.

For those providers who choose to resist program implementation, it is important to have a strategy in place to address the issue. Some programs may choose to exclude affected patients from the program because they cannot ensure physician cooperation; however, this tactic may not be appropriate for many programs. Instead, developing strategies to encourage gradual participation and working with nurses, office staff, and other caregivers as much as possible may help participants obtain the benefits of program participation despite provider reluctance.

Because physician participation in population health management strategies is usually crucial to ensure appropriate medical oversight and good quality of clinical care, overcoming potential implementation problems such as physician resistance or distrust of program sponsors is critical. When physicians resist the development of a population health management strategy because they distrust either the motivations or methodology behind the program, successful implementation may be difficult to achieve. Instead, programs designed to incorporate physician suggestions, that respond to physician criticism, and that have a basis of solid evidence from which to base estimates of program results are more likely to meet organizational goals and objectives. Establishing priorities for disease management for diseases associated with high costs or of high incidence in the target population is also important. With focus on such high-priority areas, the impact of program success is more likely to be measured and appreciated.

Further discussion of the important role of physicians in population health management is included in Chapter 13.

Prepare Staff and Physicians for Technology and Care Process Innovations

Incorporating new technologies and developing new care processes within an organization typically involves both new and existing staff in program development and implementation. Staff and physicians must be prepared to use these new tools to ensure proper population health management practices. Practitioners must be comfortable with technologies such as remote care management devices, decision support tools, and various web-based tools available to support population health management. Whether through dedicated training sessions, one-on-one feedback, or other educational strategies, the appropriate use of innovative processes and technologies must be demonstrated and learned. Chapter 14 will discuss some of the training issues surrounding the use of information technologies in further detail.

Ensure Organizational Support

As another support issue in implementation, ensuring organizational support from all levels helps to improve the likelihood of favorable program results. Ideally, inclusion of a population health management program in an organization will be consistent with the organization's mission, vision, and values. When appropriately developed based on principles of improving health and well-being while containing costs, most health management methods can be incorporated into existing organizational goals with little modification of program goals and objectives. Ensuring this goal alignment, however, is a critical consideration in program implementation.

Developing strategies to help integrate new initiatives and create program support within the organization is very important. Senior management can help support these initiatives by developing incentives for program participation and pursuing strategies such as incorporating the new program into existing efforts towards organizational change and organizational development. From a human resources perspective, a new program must be either introduced or integrated as much as possible with existing personnel to ensure good coordination and communications.

Another organizational factor that influences program implementation is organizational politics. Developing a new department or division responsible for population health management will require that department to be placed within the existing organizational hierarchy. Even for programs outsourced to vendors, determining reporting relationships and establishing accountability for program results become important considerations.

Depending, of course, on program results, the opportunities to leverage program success are plentiful. A successful program may be promoted as a key driver of future organizational success because it is an effective response to external challenges such as increasing healthcare costs and competitive pressures. Similarly, favorable outcomes may support accreditation efforts or serve as examples of quality improvement processes that work. Increases in patient satisfaction or provider satisfaction can be promoted to payers as well as potential patients and providers who will undoubtedly view such a focus with favor.

The success of population health management programs hinges largely upon the level of organizational support that can be obtained for the program. From financial commitments to visibility with senior management, the more a new program is integrated within an existing organization and is consistent with institutional goals, the better. Successful program implementation can help ensure that program goals are achieved as the organization proves able to support perceptions that the organization is both innovative and caring, lowering healthcare costs while maintaining and improving the quality of care.

Maintain Positive Organizational Culture

The introduction of a new population health management strategy can profoundly affect organizational culture. For institutions that have focused on acute care delivery or traditional approaches to case management, introduction of a population health management program that is more inclusive or integrated may be threatening. With this new strategy, institutional boundaries are no longer fixed, and physicians, care managers, and other employees are asked to consider the continuum of patient care needs regardless of setting or health status. Factors such as patient well-being, social support systems, or activities of daily living often are included in a population health management strategy that encourages healthcare personnel to work with the patient to improve health and wellness on multiple dimensions. This expanded focus necessitates a shift from an organizational culture that concentrates on delivering care only in the acute setting to a culture and care philosophy that is more patient-centered and holistic (see Table 11.2 for some of the cultural changes that can occur).

Hiring new staff has implications for organizational culture as new employees are introduced to the existing organization. However, instead of traditional approaches to acculturation that involve demonstrating and discussing organizational culture as "the way we do things around here," organizations embracing a population health management approach may be too much in flux to know what will be the best way to do things with the new philosophy. Trying to promote flexibility and acceptance of diverse thinking in any organization can smooth the culture change process that any new program development may precipitate.

Overcome Resistance to Change

As a final support issue related to program implementation, the structure and strategies of organizations may change in response to the introduction

TABLE 11.2
Cultural Changes to Promote in Population Health Management Strategy Implementation

Shift away from . . .	To consider . . .
Reactive care	Proactive assessment of health and wellness
Acute care delivery	Health and care management
Individual patients only	Individuals within populations
Patient sickness	Participant health risks and health behaviors
Traditional case management	Comprehensive care management
Fixed institutional boundaries	Continuum of care needs
Independent practitioner delivery of care	Team-based health and care management services
Specialized nurse services	Comprehensive care manager services
Fragmented service delivery	Coordinated service provision
Independent silos of financial and clinical interest	Integrated interest in population health and wellness

SOURCE: Adapted from Gurnee, M. C. and R. V. DaSilva. 1997. "Constructing Disease Management Programs." *Managed Care* [On-line article; accessed 3/3/02.] http://www.managedcaremag.com/archives/9706/9706.disease_man.shtml.

of a population health management strategy. Structural changes may be necessary to accommodate new care management departments or new employees such as care managers. New reporting relationships will emerge, and organizational politics will also be affected. When programs are outsourced to dedicated vendors, organizational structure may not change, but the importance and visibility of such programs will be evident throughout the organization. Programs that receive little attention will have little impact, but programs that are highlighted to demonstrate service and clinical improvements such as patient satisfaction, physician satisfaction, and improvements in clinical outcomes may become major strategic initiatives. Ideally, program successes will be recognized, and subsequent organizational changes may occur in response to successful program development.

Even without evident structural changes, the initiation of new programs within organizations is an obvious signal of changes taking place. And, because common responses to change are not always positive, it behooves management to recognize the unsettling nature of organizational change and develop appropriate responses to individuals' responses to change. Evidence has shown that the best approach to dealing with organizational change is to emphasize communication within the organization. By explaining what the new program is, how individuals' jobs will or will not be affected, how reporting relationships may or may not change, how expectations for performance may change, and so forth, management can help to reduce the level of uncertainty inherent in the change process. Maintaining frequent and honest communications about program progress, results, successes, and problems can help build employee awareness and, ideally, acceptance of the new program.

Organizational Theory in Practice: Organizational Change

As with many initiatives affecting management, the application of organizational theory can be very helpful in the development and implementation of population health management programs. Issues such as organizational culture, organizational structure, and organizational development are all important to consider if programs are to be successfully implemented and achieve their programmatic goals. Organizational change theories can help predict how current employees and departments will respond to the introduction of new departments or visible initiatives. Briefly considering how population health management programs can be supported.by appropriate application of organizational theories can help managers and executives to design implementation strategies and program development approaches that have the best chances of achieving success in their organizations. (See 11.4 "Organizational Change Theories" at www.ache.org/pubs/mcalearney/start.cfm.)

Strategic Control

The concept of strategic control in an organization has many facets. As described by Ginter, Swayne, and Duncan (2002), organizational controls must have certain characteristics to be effective. Organizational controls should be based on accurate, timely, and relevant information; be directed to control only critical elements; be flexible; be cost-effective; be relatively simple and easy to understand; be timely; and should emphasize exceptions overall. The framework for strategic control is cyclical and has five steps as shown in Figure 11.2. This cycle is consistent with a quality improvement cycle, and is recommended for any population health management program. Three of these elements and their importance in population health management will be described in the following sections.

Program Evaluation: Monitor Costs, Interventions, and Outcomes

Evaluating the results of a population health management strategy requires that an assessment component be incorporated into the program. This assessment becomes the basis by which program success is defined as achieved

FIGURE 11.2
Strategic
Control

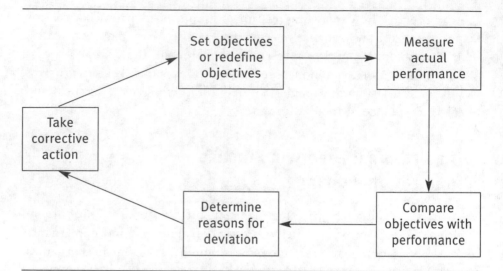

SOURCE: Adapted from: Ginter, P. M., L. E. Swayne, and W. J. Duncan. 2002. *Strategic Management of Health Care Organizations*. Malden, MA: Blackwell Publishers.

or not. Considering the program outcomes perspective of interest (as described in Chapter 4) will help narrow or broaden the focus of the program evaluation.

From initial selection of program goals to overall evaluation of program success, outcomes definition and measurement are critical. Population health management programs can be evaluated from multiple perspectives, and given the perspectives of these various parties, different outcomes may be an appropriate focus. One major distinction in outcomes research is between short-term and long-term outcomes. Program sponsors responsible for program costs and savings may be interested in achieving cost reduction goals as quickly as possible. However, from the standpoint of the main beneficiaries of health management programs—the patients—it is vital to maintain a strong program focus on long-term outcomes such as quality of life and health improvement. A lifestyle management approach using a smoking cessation program to decrease tobacco use may have as one of its stated goals "to reduce the number of smokers in a population." The true health outcome, however, may be a reduction in cases of heart disease and lung cancer and overall reduced morbidity for this population.

Collecting baseline utilization data is critical for program evaluation. Information can be collected about bed day utilization, number of hospitalizations, number of emergency department visits, number of outpatient visits, and so forth, depending on the outcomes of interest, and can draw from a variety of databases and utilization surveys. Additional preliminary data collection for participants focused on clinical and biologic measurements such as height, weight, blood pressure, and laboratory values will require clinical assessment but will also provide invaluable information about the baseline health status of program participants. Often, using health assessments of some sort in either the population selection process or in program initiation can provide a baseline from which to measure improvements or changes in population health. Specifically, questions regarding functional health status, perceived health status, emotional well-being, and modifiable health risk behaviors will help programs track progress made against such metrics. Other metrics that may also be important for program evaluation purposes are process measures. Tracking metrics such as appointment waiting times for clinical visits, time spent on hold for telephonic demand management services, or time spent with patients by various providers enables program developers to monitor service to clients and program costs. Finally, in considering the additional outcomes of interest to program sponsors such as health plans or employers, tracking metrics such as per-member-per-month costs, member turnover, physician and patient satisfaction, employee absenteeism, employer disability costs, and other outcomes are important.

The careful design of program evaluations structured to provide evidence of health management program progress and success is very important. To facilitate this process, including evaluation specialists such as health services researchers, health economists, or biostatisticians as program personnel may be beneficial. These individuals will be able to provide oversight for the development of program evaluations of appropriate size and design. Such professional expertise can also help program developers focus on the importance of various outcomes perspectives and emphasize the need to collect different types of healthcare, utilization, and survey data. Taking time during program design and implementation to define outcomes of interest and determine how to measure and track such outcomes can help improve program focus and results. This careful consideration at the design stage of a program is vital to ensure that a population health management program's achievements are both measurable and irrefutable.

Evaluate Participant Satisfaction

Ensuring participant satisfaction with population health management programs is also crucial. Employers want their employees to be satisfied with the services offered, just as hospitals and other providers want patients to be satisfied with their care. Similarly, health management programs want participants to be satisfied with program services, as well as with the clinical and programmatic outcomes.

Measurement of program satisfaction may rely on standard satisfaction survey tools, or more specialized instruments may need to be developed. In many situations, information about employee, patient, or member satisfaction is already being collected. Existing information can be used as a baseline from which to measure any improvements or decrements in satisfaction and to ensure that program satisfaction goals are being met.

However, the disadvantage of relying only on existing tools such as standard patient satisfaction surveys is that any changes in patient satisfaction may or may not be directly attributable to the implementation of a health management program. It may be impossible to disentangle the reasons for observed changes.

An alternative approach is to develop a program-specific satisfaction tool that addresses similar participant satisfaction concerns but concentrates on the population health management program. By administering such a tool prior to program implementation and then following up with program participants to remeasure satisfaction at fixed time intervals, it is more likely that changes can be linked to program results. More importantly, by including questions that address program factors specifically—such as satisfaction with care managers, accessibility of information, or helpfulness of educational materials—these program components can be directly assessed.

Incorporate Quality Improvement

Including a quality improvement component within population health management programs ensures that programs are developed and refined using the best available evidence. Quality improvement processes and methodologies are, in fact, consistent with the approaches to health management discussed in this text. In particular, the notion of continuous improvement in the plan-do-check-act (PDCA) cycle is important to include in population health management programs that attempt to improve health and well-being on an ongoing basis. Ideally, programs are planned, then implemented, and then their results checked by some sort of evaluation. When evidence is not strong that the program is making a difference, programs need to either initiate a cycle of redesign, or consider dramatic modifications to ensure that they attain their objectives.

While formal continuous quality improvement (CQI) or total quality management (TQM) training is not necessary, the recommended step of building an evaluation component into the design stage of a program is consistent with these approaches. Given the importance of good program outcomes and the need to produce solid evidence to support program continuation or expansion, it is wise to keep the notion of continuous improvement in mind.

In practice, population health management programs may be adopted by healthcare organizations as a part of their own quality improvement strategies. When faced with accreditation requirements from NCQA or JCAHCO, organizations may discover that developing a population health management program helps them set measurable quality improvement goals for the health of their members or patients and also to devise a plan to work towards those goals. As an example, a disease management program offered through a health plan may increase the number of preventive health screenings for a given population, as recommended by NCQA guidelines.

Keeping in mind the goals of quality improvement in the context of improvements in both health and healthcare quality can help guide programs from their initiation. Whether a program is built in-house or purchased from an outside company, quality improvement goals can clarify program and sponsor expectations. By selecting measurable outcomes that are consistent with health management program objectives, a quality improvement framework can help emphasize the importance of ongoing measurement and program refinements in the context of health improvement.

Conclusion

The introduction of population health management strategies into an organization has a number of implications for management. Population health management program development may require major changes of organizational strategy, structure, and culture. Implementation may be more challenging because of the need to obtain employee and physician acceptance of new program strategies. Innovative care processes and technologies may require new skills and attitudes. A strategic program management focus can facilitate implementation and ongoing management by aligning population health management goals with organizational goals and values. Considering some of the important service delivery, support, and strategic control issues as described in this chapter can smooth the program implementation process because new initiatives will not be perceived as being at cross purposes with existing organizational plans. By promoting improvements in clinical and financial outcomes, well-implemented population health management strategies can help realize the overall health policy goals of better individual and population health.

REFERENCES

Bodenheimer, T. 1999. "Disease Management—Promises and Pitfalls." *New England Journal of Medicine* 340 (15): 1202–05.

Buelow, J. O. 2002. Personal communication, February.

Ginter, P. M., L. E. Swayne, and W. J. Duncan. 2002. *Strategic Management of Health Care Organizations*. Malden, MA: Blackwell Publishers.

Gurnee, M. C. and R. V. DaSilva. 1997. "Constructing Disease Management Programs." *Managed Care*. [On-line article; accessed 3/3/02.] http://www.managedcaremag.com/archives/9706/9706.disease_man.shtml.

Herzlinger, R. 1997. *Market Driven Healthcare*. Reading, MA: Addison-Wesley Publishing Company.

Hodges, L. C., J. C. Hall-Barrow, and T. C. Satkowski. 1998. "Chronic Disease Management Offers New Career Opportunities." *MedSurg Nursing* 4 (7): 228–35.

McAlearney, A. S. 2002. "Population Health Management in Theory and Practice." In *Advances in Health Care Management* (Volume 3), edited by G. T. Savage, J. Blair, and M. Fottler. New York: JAI Press/ Elsevier Science Ltd.

McAlearney, A. S. 2000. "Designing and Developing Effective Disease Management Programmes: Key Decisions for Programme Success." *Disease Management and Health Outcomes* 7 (3): 139–48.

Porter, M. E. 1985. *Competitive Advantage: Creating and Sustaining Superior Performance*. New York: Free Press.

Ritterband, D. R. 2000. "Disease Management: Old Wine in New Bottles?" *Journal of Healthcare Management* 45 (4): 255–66.

Schmidt, J. 2000. "Key Issues to Ponder when Designing Your DM Program." The Managed Care Information Center. [On-line article; accessed 5/14/01.] https://wwws.monmouth.com/themcic/ac-odm.htm.

Skinner, W. 1974. "The Focused Factory." *Harvard Business Review* (May–Jun): 113–22.

CARE MANAGERS

For many population health management approaches, a critical player in the clinical area is some type of care manager. In practice, care managers may have a variety of titles including case manager, nurse manager, care coordinator, program coordinator, or health educator. The 2001 International Case/Care Management Conference acknowledged the level of ambiguity in the title care or case manager because these "overlapping terms used in different countries and health settings—have become international buzzwords that signify such wide-ranging ideas as consumer choice, potential cost savings to government health systems hoping to control expensive cases, or the hiring of private care managers for a family elder" (Kleyman 2001).

In the context of this book, the common function of care managers is to provide integrative care management services for patients or members participating in a population health management program. This chapter will present some of the issues surrounding the critical role care managers play in population health management and describe various human resources concerns related to the hiring, training, and retaining of care managers in population health management practice.

Types of Care Managers

A broad range of clinical specialists can be defined as care managers for population health management programs. Beyond physicians (discussed in Chapter 13), care managers may include nurses, social workers, counselors, educators, and other ancillary therapists. Most frequently, care managers in health management programs are nurses. Programs typically try to recruit registered nurses to ensure the quality of their clinical services and help avoid questions about the appropriateness of their care managers' recommendations. These nurses may provide direct patient care services or may be exclusively available over the telephone, depending on program focus, as illustrated in Table 12.1.

In addition to nurses, population health management programs may use other types of practitioners as care managers. For programs that attempt to address both physical and mental health issues, it is important to have care managers with appropriate skill sets to cover the range of potential patient problems. Social workers, for example, serve well as care managers for population health management programs that especially focus on

TABLE 12.1
Care Managers
in Practice

Types	Settings	Roles
Physicians	• Office practice • Hospital • Clinic	• Provision of care • Coordination of care • Clinical oversight
Nurses	• Office practice • Hospital • Clinic • Remote location (telephonic) • Patient home	• Guidance and advice • Provision of care in physician office, hospital, clinic • Home-based care
Social Workers	• Office practice • Hospital • Clinic • Remote location (telephonic) • Patient home	• Guidance and advice • Assistance with social and personal concerns • Home-based services • Arrangement of services
Counselors (including psychologists, psychotherapists)	• Office practice • Hospital • Clinic • Remote location (telephonic) • Employer site	• Counseling • Behavior modification therapy
Educators	• Office • Hospital • Clinic • Remote location (telephonic) • Employer site	• Educational advice and guidance • Assistance with behavior change advice and protocols
Nutritionists	• Office • Hospital • Clinic • Remote location (telephonic) • Employer site	• Guidance and advice • Assistance with behavior change advice and protocols

providing a range of social and behavioral support services. Programs that work beyond the acute-care setting to offer social support within a community setting may rely on social workers who are familiar with community agencies and organizations that can be of assistance to participating patients.

Health management programs with a strong behavioral health component may have specialists such as psychologists or psychotherapists defined as care managers to serve as counselors for participants. For example, a disease management program focused on depression may benefit from having a combination of clinical and behavioral health experts as part of a care management team. Similarly, a disability management program concerned about mental health may enlist the help of behavioral healthcare managers to provide specialized support in mental and behavioral health issues.

Health educators and nurse educators comprise another category of care managers for health management programs. When educating patients about the progress and treatment of chronic diseases is a central component of a program, these health educators serve as primary care managers for a good portion of the population health management program. Diabetes disease management programs, for example, often rely on diabetes nurse educators to counsel patients about their modifiable health risks and behavioral choices. Such programs recruit ancillary clinician educators such as nutritionists to focus on issues related to diabetes control including diet and weight management.

Offering the proper mix of direct clinical providers and supporting clinicians and counselors is very important for all population health management programs. Appropriate provider selection and involvement can help programs to best manage program resources and capabilities. Furthermore, by providing patients with access to a wide range of care managers to help them better manage their health, these programs become part of an empowerment process for involved participants that can, ultimately, help them improve their own health status.

Settings and Functions

Care managers function in a variety of settings: through telephone contact with enrolled patients, through computer-assisted monitoring, or through face-to-face contacts if home- or office-based services are a major program component. A common arrangement for many population health management programs is to have a care manager who functions mainly from an outpatient, nonhospital setting; however, many variations are possible. Demand management programs typically offer telephonic services such as advice and counseling and retain care managers who have no expectations for direct patient care. When clinical services are required for demand management program participants, care managers can use a referral list of appropriate providers to obtain necessary care for their patients. Care managers in lifestyle management programs might similarly offer telephone-based advice and support to promote health behavior change and improvements in participant risk behaviors and well-being without expecting substantial direct participant contact.

Disease management programs typically employ care managers who interact with patients on multiple levels. Telephone-based contact may form the basis for most patient care interactions, and, depending on the sophistication of the program, computer-based communications may also be important. In more involved programs care managers may be used to make direct clinical assessments of enrolled patients. These programs may send care managers to evaluate new patients in their own houses and may also have associated follow-up visits, when appropriate.

Care managers in catastrophic care management programs function similarly to care managers in disease management programs, but many of their nonclinical activities are related to coordination of care. Telephone-based contact with multiple providers and involved family members can form the basis of their patient-related activities while they manage the health and rehabilitation of their patient participants. Disability management programs have care managers employed from the employer side who are responsible for managing the program and employees covered in a disability program. These individuals often work from the employer's offices and are responsible for establishing contact with and monitoring the needs of employees according to their situations. Alternatively, disability management services may be offered through insurance companies or be outsourced to private companies. In these situations, care managers provide similar services even though their employment is external to the contracting employer.

While less common for population health management programs, care managers can also have their primary function in the inpatient setting. In contrast to hospital-based clinicians such as traditional case managers or hospitalist physicians, care managers are most likely to focus on issues related to post-discharge care and follow-up. As they coordinate services that have been initiated from a hospital stay, they often are responsible for some discharge planning, as well as coordination of any post-acute care services needed. While direct patient service is naturally incorporated into these care managers' initial contacts with their clients in the hospital, follow-up activities, similar to other programs, typically emphasize fewer clinical visits and more remote care management.

Care Manager Roles

Given the wide variety of types of care managers, it is no surprise that they have many jobs to perform. From telephone calls to home visits to counseling to education, care managers are charged with the broad task of helping patients to improve their health and well-being. In practice, the tasks performed by care managers vary by program type as well as by type of care manager. Traditionally, care management functions include the following:

- identifying high-risk patients to be served;
- performing assessments;
- developing care plans, using protocols if indicated;
- facilitating access to medical and social services;

- coordinating services;
- monitoring services and the care plan (i.e., monitoring health status, improvements, progress of care protocol); and
- measuring and evaluating outcomes.

Formal definitions of case or care management emphasize the importance of comprehensive services provided across an entire illness episode for a patient, regardless of location of service or type of payment. Overall, care or case management needs to be organized, interdisciplinary, and coordinated with respect to clinical, quality, and financial management issues (Satinsky 1995).

In the context of population health management, care managers are expected to play a number of roles in most programs. Particularly important roles for care managers, regardless of the actual label, include the following:

- care coordination;
- individual identification and assessment;
- promoting health improvement;
- coordination with providers;
- data collection; and
- communication and collaboration.

Care Coordination

For many population health management programs, one care manager serves as the primary point of contact for a number of individual patients. These programs encourage collaboration among multiple care managers with different areas of expertise, but a primary care manager is typically responsible for overall coordination and oversight of a particular group of patients. This central care manager ensures that patients do not experience any gaps in service and keeps track of the patients' progress towards population health management program goals.

The general care coordination function is especially important in population health management programs focused on specific diseases or conditions. Given the nature of most diseases selected for disease management, multiple referrals to multiple providers may not be well coordinated. Worse, multiple visits can overwhelm the patient with an overload of information that can be confusing or even contradictory. The care coordination role in such situations is clearly critical. When a nurse functions in this care manager role, she or he can help to filter information that the patient receives. The care manager can also assist the patient by keeping the larger clinical picture in mind, trying to avoid gaps in care or missed services that the patient may not be able to track. Having a care manager to manage the care process can organize and rationalize the provision of services from multiple providers who may or may not communicate with each other or with the patient. The care manager's role in such situations is to coordinate such communications while also helping the patient to understand the progress of his or her treatment.

Another important element of care coordination is in organizing different types of care management services. In the case of a disease complicated by comorbidities or other complex management issues, optimal health management may require involvement of multiple types of care managers. For some cases, it is conceivable that one patient would be expected to receive health management assistance from a nurse, a social worker, an educator, and a nutritionist, all in the name of good disease management. Coordination of these multiple care managers, both with respect to ensuring that they make contact with the patient and that the patient understands their recommendations, must also fall to the primary care manager. It is important that the patient feel that he or she is truly in the center of the health management equation and that all the appropriate contacts are made and understood.

Individual Identification and Assessment

As described in Chapter 4 on targeting individuals for population health management, many methods exist by which to identify populations and individuals for care management interventions. In practice, care managers can play an important role in this targeting process, especially when surveys or assessments are included as part of the process of identifying individuals for intervention. Care managers may help directly with the survey or assessment process or provide professional expertise with follow-up assessments to ensure that individuals identified based on other types of data and analysis are actually appropriate for program inclusion. When it is possible to make personal contact with target individuals, care managers can further apply screening criteria to the defined population selected to ensure appropriate targeting.

After individuals are identified for inclusion in population health management programs, care managers play a vital role in performing various assessments. Initial assessments may be based on health risk or health habits, followed by detailed assessments depending on diseases or conditions. A dynamic assessment process is very important to ensure that the population health management program is both current in the information it uses and accurate in the information it collects (Nash 2000). Care managers can facilitate dynamic assessment by performing follow-up assessments at prescribed intervals, by maintaining ongoing contact and communications with target individuals, and by keeping current with treatment guidelines and protocols so that appropriate care patterns are followed. When the health status of an individual changes either because of intervention or acute care need, care managers can monitor these changes and modify care plans as necessary.

Promoting Health Improvement

In addition to the broad care coordination function expected of most care managers, population health management programs typically have some sort of health improvement agenda that care managers are expected to lead. Whether in the form of direct patient care and counseling or in providing education and treatment support, care managers play a vital role in fulfilling program goals related to health improvement.

The role of care managers in promoting health improvement is particularly evident when they participate in patient education. Disease management programs often take advantage of the value of group educational settings and include activities such as support groups for diabetics or CHF patients led by care managers. Regularly scheduled group meetings can be used to both provide social support for participants and set an educational schedule of topics related to disease management and health improvement. Catastrophic care management programs and disease management programs focused on chronic illnesses also rely on care managers as they use the program as an opportunity to educate family members and other caregivers about the diseases and their sequelae. By including the patient's support network in the education process, patients ideally receive more assistance from those individuals because of their increased understanding of the importance of modifying risky health behaviors and following through with appropriate self-care plans.

Demand management programs may also leverage the role of care managers in promoting health improvement. In some demand management programs, nurses follow strict algorithms or decision rules to guide patients to make appropriate medical care utilization decisions. However, other programs may be focused on an individual program initiative such as emphasizing appropriate referrals to specialists, and they can use incoming phone calls as an opportunity to educate members about both their clinical conditions and their options to access the healthcare system. More intensive programs supplement care manager responses to incoming calls with outbound calls to participants to discuss topics related to health improvement initiatives underway. Schedules may even be set for outbound calls to patients when health education topics can be discussed. As an example, programs with a lifestyle management component such as a smoking cessation strategy can include formalized schedules of calls for care managers to make to participants educating them about their health risks, encouraging them to change their behaviors, and celebrating their progress towards their goals.

From a clinical perspective, disease management programs often focus specifically on clinical health improvements such as reductions in blood pressure or cholesterol as they help patients manage their chronic illnesses. In such programs, care managers are able to track member progress towards health improvement goals by checking available laboratory and clinical data as patients have visits with various providers. More sophisticated programs that rely heavily on information technologies enable nurses to monitor participant blood pressure, weight, or blood sugar remotely via computer or telephonic entries recorded by the patients themselves. This clinical oversight helps ensure that any worrisome laboratory value is checked and that enrolled patients are appropriately followed by clinical personnel.

Another important function of care managers in the context of promoting health improvement is to educate staff and other members of the care management team about health improvement. By keeping team members up to date about the progress of care plans, health improvement goals, and any barriers to success, care managers can improve the intervention process and facilitate health improvement in their patients. Members of the care team may be motivated to further promote health among program clients, increasing the likelihood of program success.

Finally, care managers play an important role in educating patients and their families to be their own care managers. As self-care opportunities are promoted through all population health management strategies, care managers become an important conduit for this education and training. Helping to develop the abilities of patients to care for themselves, define quality in ways that are appropriate for these individuals (Geron 2001), and make healthy decisions about their behaviors become critical tasks for program care managers.

Coordination with Physician Providers

Another vital role for all care managers is in promoting coordination with physician providers. Especially in situations where disease or condition management is characterized by multiple physician visits, care managers are charged to help coordinate care among multiple visits and multiple providers. Even when physician visits are infrequent, care managers play an important role by updating the physician about what has happened to individual patients since their last visits.

Best practices in population health management are characterized by strong involvement of physician providers in most aspects of program design and implementation (as described in Chapter 11 and Chapter 13). Physicians may continue to provide an oversight role in the program, but the daily responsibility for monitoring patient progress with respect to health management issues usually falls to care managers. Care managers must remain aware of physician preferences regarding involvement in their patients' care and alert those providers about any clinical changes. Further, in many programs, documentation of all care management patient contacts must be provided for the patients' primary care physicians so that such information is retained in the medical records.

The coordination role of care managers is central to keeping providers informed about their patients' progress and ensuring the best possible clinical care for those individuals. This role also keeps patients informed about their providers' needs and expectations for their clinical visits. By maintaining good contact with both physicians and population health management program participants, care managers help realize program goals of improved patient understanding and health status, and increased provider satisfaction.

Data Collection

Care managers are also expected to collect data and maintain documentation about participating patients in population health management programs. Similar to data and reporting requirements in other areas of healthcare, data collection is vitally important for population health management programs. Good documentation ensures oversight of clinical care and health management program processes. Patients who are enrolled in such programs benefit from dedicated clinical oversight and a level of quality assurance that is important for all such endeavors.

Documentation also helps care managers of all types keep track of the needs and preferences of program participants. Especially in programs where patients can visit multiple providers and multiple care managers, maintaining documentation and data about patient contacts ensures that care provided is consistent and directed towards common health improvement goals. Furthermore, when patients are handed off from one provider to the next, the receiving provider can have access to the overall picture of patient care and contacts to quickly and logically determine the next steps for this patient.

Data collection is clearly critical from a quality improvement perspective. Research projects trying to improve quality in care or service rely on data collected to document both starting and ending points, and attempts to evaluate care processes in a health management program rely on careful documentation of those processes. If waiting times are a problem, for example, such waiting times must be recorded, and care managers may be responsible for making sure that the data collected are both thorough and accurate. Showing evidence of improvements is only possible if documentation exists, and the burden of ensuring that such data are collected often falls to care managers who are centrally involved in the programs being assessed.

Finally, data collection is important because of its central role in outcomes research. From beginning steps in baseline data collection to later progress reports and aggregate analysis, data must be collected in a systematic and organized fashion. Many programs rely upon standardized surveys and questionnaires to capture information about factors such as disease status or the presence of social support systems. However, the results of these surveys are usually interpreted by clinicians such as care managers and may indicate a need for patient follow-up. These more detailed health assessments are typically completed by care managers. Even when data collection methodologies are largely computer-based, it is incumbent upon care managers or their associates to enter those data and make sure that participants provide answers to the questions asked.

Although the importance of this data collection role should not surprise care managers, the need to use automated data collection systems in many population health management programs may be intimidating. Good programs take these requirements into account in their hiring and training processes to ensure that data collection can proceed reliably under the guidance of committed care managers. This emphasis helps ensure that data collected are reliable, valid, and sufficient to provide evidence of good service and care quality, program achievements, and participant satisfaction.

Communication

With all population health management programs, the importance of communication is clear. Good patient communication skills are vital to understanding and addressing patient needs. Good communication with patients' family members and other caregivers also extends the reach of health management programs in the best interest of those patients. Communication with providers is also clearly important. Beyond coordinating physician and care manager activities, maintaining open lines of communication assists both patients and health management programs.

From a physician perspective, a major challenge of many population health management programs is that not all of their patients are enrolled in the same program. Instead, a physician must often work with multiple programs associated with the variety of health plan contracts and employer programs connected to his or her patients. They may have to deal with multiple disease treatment algorithms or care protocols, different care manager report formats, and a variety of expectations for provider involvement depending on which program is relevant to a particular patient. Even following standard treatment guidelines may not be sufficient to comply with specific disease management program protocols designed for an individual insurer. In such situations, it is imperative that the care manager understands the vital communication role that is expected of her or him. Making clear expectations about two-way communications between providers and the program as well as three-way communications that also involve the patient is usually the responsibility of the care manager. Care managers must be able to communicate about other program needs such as data collection, quality, and collaboration.

Collaboration

Also crucial in population health management is collaboration. For individuals who receive services from multiple types of care managers, collaboration is critical to ensure clinical needs are addressed as well as social and behavioral concerns. Care managers cannot work at cross purposes, and patient needs must be kept central in any programmatic decisions.

The collaborative role of care managers is especially important in the context of those programs which leverage the use of services available in the community. Patient participants may benefit greatly from opportunities presented by nonprogram services that supplement program offerings such as meals on wheels, respite care, or durable medical equipment loans or rentals. It is important that care managers remain aware of available community services and be willing to work with external service providers.

Care manager collaboration is also important from a program perspective. To the extent that multiple health management programs exist within the same provider's office or even for the same patient who suffers from multiple health problems, the care manager must take responsibility for rationalizing care and service processes. Care managers play an important role in reducing service duplication and improving patient understanding of clinical advice. Furthermore, care managers must ensure that both patients and providers understand health improvement goals and the steps necessary to improve both health and well-being.

Finally, collaboration with program sponsors may be another relevant concern. When employers are involved in program design or are concerned about program results, employer representatives may expect to be contacted regularly about program progress and employee activities. Similarly, programs sponsored by health plans often designate a health plan representative to oversee a health management initiative, and care managers may be responsible for keeping such individuals informed about both the positive and negative aspects of the program.

When problems arise with either participants or providers, it is helpful for care managers to be in contact with program sponsors or directors to resolve such issues. Similarly, challenges such as resource allocation, inadequate training of personnel, or insufficient information systems capabilities are more easily addressed if collaborative relationships exist with program sponsors. Care managers who are sensitive to such programmatic concerns are more likely to receive needed organizational support, whether financial or human resources, to help their efforts.

Human Resources Issues

Selecting and training individuals to be care managers for population health management programs poses an organizational challenge. Integrating these care managers into an existing organization can present further challenges. Turf issues and concerns about political power and control may emerge with the addition of new staff and a new program. Whether care managers are new hires or are brought into an organization as part of a contract with an outside vendor, the incorporation of those individuals into the existing organization can be problematic. Similarly, when a health management program receives substantial visibility and focus, this may lead to issues such as rivalry with existing programs and conflicts among employees.

Human resources issues must be addressed whether a program is built in-house or outsourced to a contracted vendor. Especially because of the multiple roles care managers must play, challenges such as hiring the right personnel, offering appropriate training for new hires and program participants, and retaining good care managers are to be expected.

Hiring

Depending on the type of care manager needed, hiring can be difficult, if not impossible. When nurses are required, the short supply of nurses in different geographic areas becomes a considerable problem. However, the care management position presents new career opportunities for many healthcare professionals. For nurses interested in shifting their focus from 100-percent patient care to a wider variety of tasks, the opportunity to work as a care manager may be well received. Demand management programs, in particular, offer flexible and varied work schedules that are manageable for nurses and other types of care managers. Disease management programs provide a good balance of direct patient contact with the opportunity to explore new areas such as program development, management, or outcomes research. Providing such opportunities within the care manager job description may help expand the pool of interested applicants for such positions.

Selecting appropriate individuals for the care manager job, however, is not easy. For clinical providers accustomed to narrowly defined work roles and face-to-face contact with patients, the care manager position presents a new set of challenges. Individuals who will succeed in the care manager role must be flexible and comfortable with constant change. Population health management programs are rarely stagnant, so care managers must be able to adapt to ongoing program refinements and modifications.

It is also very important that each care manager possess the clinical skills necessary to do the defined job. Whether nursing, counseling, or educating, care managers typically work very independently with little program oversight. In many program environments, care managers are expected to work within general program guidelines and may be held accountable for the progress and outcomes of their patients. When problems arise, it is incumbent upon care managers to seek necessary guidance, whether clinical or programmatic, and devise solutions largely on their own. Successful care managers thrive with this level of autonomy and independence, achieving program goals for their patients' health improvement while focusing on both quality and efficiency concerns.

Care managers must also be comfortable with technology. Whether existing programs are largely paper-based or computer-driven, future enhancements will certainly lead towards greater reliance on information technology. Successful care managers will need to be comfortable learning new technologies and helping others, including patients, to also become comfortable with such systems. The ability of care managers to help with program design in areas such as adaptation for technology enhancements or even computer program or software design—especially since programs constantly grow and change—can be very valuable. Potential care managers interested in developing these skills will find that most health management programs offer a wide range of such opportunities.

Finally, care managers must possess excellent communication skills and an ability to work with multiple types of people. From direct patient contact to communications with physicians, care managers must be able to clearly communicate their message and stand up for the needs of their patients and the goals of their program. Such skill in communication will facilitate achievement of desired program outcomes including improved health and well-being for program participants.

Training and Development

In human resources, employee training is but one step in a continuum of activities designed to develop care managers. This continuum proceeds from the concepts of initial orientation training, skills training, and in-service education to include additional development activities such as continuing education and career development (Smith and Fottler 1998).

Training and development programs for care managers can be comprehensive or ad hoc, depending on the nature of the population health management program being staffed. Care managers who join health management programs from full-time clinical care positions often require less training about expectations for clinical care activities, but may be unfamiliar with the requirements and expectations of such programs. Initial training and orientation should be designed to introduce employees to organizational values, mores, beliefs, behaviors, standard operating procedures, policies, and expectations (Smith & Fottler 1998) associated with the specific population health management program. Orientation training should focus on how to use required information technologies, how to represent oneself as a care manager in the context of the population health management program, and how to work with participating providers. Additional training may proceed depending on the individual requirements and emphases of different population health management programs.

For demand management programs, much of the program content is contained in the algorithms or decision rules care managers are expected to follow when they answer the telephone for client calls. Learning how these algorithms work and learning what flexibility is—or more importantly, is not—expected is an important component of care manager training. Skill training usually consists of multiple hours of supervised telephone calls to assess a care manager's ability to provide consistent and understandable advice over the telephone. Care managers must also be able to respond appropriately to callers' spontaneous and unexpected questions. Most demand management programs rely on care managers to make appropriate referrals to physicians or other providers, so training may also consist of familiarizing care managers with the providers available to serve their client base.

Training for disease management programs, similar to that for demand management programs, usually begins with care managers learning the content of the specific program. Care managers hired for programs in cardiovascular disease, for example, usually have some experience caring for persons with the disease, but they must learn the particular program format and guidelines they are expected to follow. In addition to overall clinical training, care managers will typically be introduced to their role in data collection and outcomes research. They will receive training about the various surveys and assessments they must complete or have their patients complete, and they will learn what to do with the data they obtain.

Care managers can also be expected to keep track of programmatic information for the purposes of calculating program costs and benefits. Measures such as the time spent with different clients, performing certain tasks, and coordinating care and information with providers may all be tracked to determine cost per client or cost per change in patient outcome. Some programs also assess the value of care management activities by defining softer outcomes such as provider visits averted or hospital stays avoided. Although these metrics may not provide hard evidence to justify program success, keeping track of such information supplements anecdotal evidence of the effect of care managers and the program on their patient population.

Additional training requirements for care managers will depend on the specific type of population health management program being staffed. Programs with an emphasis on rare diseases or catastrophic conditions will spend a considerable amount of training resources to help care managers understand most aspects of the disease and implications of the disease for patients, their families, and their lives. In contrast, programs focused mainly on lifestyle management will concentrate training on how to improve care managers' abilities to encourage client behavior change by working with behavioral concepts such as "readiness and willingness to change" behavior as described in Prochaska's transtheoretical model of behavior change (Prochaska et al. 1992; 1994; Prochaska and Velicer 1997).

Care manager training can also include basic management skills training to teach care managers how to work with the different types of support staff they may encounter. In addition to personal management skills such as time management or dealing with change, skill development can include instruction in how to run effective meetings, how to obtain collaboration among differently trained individuals, and how to work with data to develop reports and track client progress towards outcomes. Communication skills training can be added to enhance those skills in the context of a health management program, as well as to strengthen skills in the areas of provider and patient relations.

Another component of training programs should be a retraining schedule for care managers. As new protocols are included in a demand management program or new diseases are added for management, care managers should be expected to participate in comprehensive in-service educational programs to improve their skill sets. The incorporation of new technologies or new data collection strategies provides another opportunity for retraining. Periodic assessment of care manager skills and patient management abilities should be included in any training program to guarantee quality on a continual basis for population health management programs. Developing a thorough and ongoing training program for care managers can ensure that personnel hired for population health management programs are equipped with the appropriate skills and competencies to best serve both patients and sponsoring organizations.

Finally, considering the overarching goal of career development for care managers, it is important to move beyond skills training and organizational acculturation. Career development plans should help expand staff capabilities in a dynamic educational process. Ideally, care management programs should provide the background for development of a comprehensive set of skills much broader than the traditional professional domains from which care managers are drawn. Incorporating training in information systems, data management, and outcomes research provides opportunities for care managers to expand their professional competencies to areas they may decide to later pursue. Similarly, helping care managers to grow personally by supporting them with management skills training or communications programs is also mutually beneficial to employees and the organization. By attempting to integrate individual and organizational goals for overall employee development, population health management programs will attract and support excellent care managers committed to the goals of population health improvement.

Retention

In addition to the recruitment, hiring, training, and development of good care managers, a key human resources function for any organization is to focus on employee retention. For care managers whose skill sets or goals are incompatible with program goals, early dismissal may be appropriate. However, it is important to retain and satisfy well-trained and high-performing care managers. After care manager training in population health management functions, individual marketability improves, and these care managers gain a broader perspective about the careers that are appropriate and possible for them to consider, making an organizational focus on retention critical.

Employee turnover is linked to how satisfied individuals are with both their organization and their job (Landau and Abelson 1998).

Specifically, the more commitment people feel towards the organization and the more their personal goals and values match those of the organization, the more likely they are to remain with that organization (Mowday et al. 1982). Developing an environment that fosters such organizational commitment is critical for a population health management program. For many clinical professionals, values alignment is facilitated by focusing on patient concerns and patient health improvement. Because the goals of population health management programs are consistent with a patient-centered model of care as well as a focus on care quality and health improvement, dedicated clinical professionals should see goal alignment with the program. However, for programs that overemphasize cost containment or efficiency over concerns about patients and health improvements, goal alignment is likely to be difficult. Such misalignment will create employee dissatisfaction and can lead to care manager turnover.

Multiple stages are identifiable in the turnover process (Mobley 1977). Satisfaction with one's position is the desired first stage, and this is influenced by various psychological, individual, organizational, and environmental factors. The second stage of turnover involves thinking about leaving one's position. This stage may be influenced by job dissatisfaction (Porter & Steers 1973), as well as by issues such as awareness of opportunities elsewhere (March & Simon 1958), or because friends and colleagues have left or are considering leaving (Krackhardt and Porter 1985).

In turnover's third stage, individuals search for alternative employment opportunities. For nurses and other clinicians who have been well trained as care managers, these alternative opportunities can be numerous. Not only can care managers find employment with other population health management programs, they also have opportunities related to the skills they have developed on the job. Personnel who were formerly exclusively clinical often discover an aptitude for information systems or healthcare management, and they can leverage the experience they have had as care managers to find new positions.

In the fourth stage of turnover, employees compare alternatives with their present position and make a decision; in the fifth stage, they actually leave or stay (Mobley 1977). Greater search activities on the part of an employee may make his or her leaving more probable, but it may only take one favorable opportunity to spark the decision to leave. Program management must be aware of the issues surrounding the turnover decision process so that they can attempt to influence their employees' decisions, if this is possible and desirable.

Most turnover is considered dysfunctional because retained employees would be defined as competent high-performers who are difficult to replace. Keeping an eye on the market to ensure that salaries remain competitive and attractive, providing good working conditions and a positive organizational culture, and making sure that the population health management program's reputation and outcomes are as positive as possible are all within the purview of good program managers. These steps create a good working environment where excellent care managers will be motivated to stay and perform.

Conclusion

As described in this chapter, the role of the care manager in any population health management program is critical. Regardless of professional background, good care managers must be recruited, developed, and appreciated. The multiple roles they play range from care coordination to data collection to communication—and they must all be executed with excellence. It is vital that health management programs recognize the centrality and importance of these care managers and work to hire and retain those with values and goals congruent with program goals. By maintaining this focus on good employees, a population health management program can have the best chance possible of succeeding in its efforts to improve health and well-being for both individuals and a population.

REFERENCES

Geron, S. M. 2001. "The Quality of Consumer-directed Long-term Care." *Generations* 24 (3): 66. [On-line article; accessed 2/2202.] http://www.asaging.org/generations/gen-24-3/qualitycons.html.

Kleyman, P. 2001. "Care Management: Who Wants It, Who Gets It, Does It Work?" *Aging Today* (Sept./October). [On-line article; accessed 1/22/02.] http://www.asaging.org/at/at-221/CareManage.html.

Krackhardt, D., and L. W. Porter. 1985. "When Friends Leave: A Structural Analysis of the Relationship Between Turnover and Stayers' Attitudes." *Administrative Science Quarterly* 30 (2): 242–61.

Landau, J., and M. Abelson. 1998. "Recruitment and Retention." In *Essentials of Human Resources Management in Health Services Organizations*, edited by M. Fottler, S. R. Hernandez, and C. L. Joiner. Albany, NY: Delmar Publishers.

March, J. G., and H. A. Simon. 1958. *Organizations*. New York: Wiley.

Mobley, W. H. 1977. "Intermediate Linkages in the Relationship Between Job Satisfaction and Employee Turnover." *Journal of Applied Psychology* 62 (2): 237–40.

Mowday, R. T., L. W. Porter, and R. M. 1982. *Employee-Organizational Linkages: The Psychology of Commitment, Absenteeism, and Turnover* New York: Academic Press.

Nash, I. S. 2000. "Dynamic Assessment in Disease Management." *Disease Management and Health Outcomes* 8 (3): 139–46.

Porter, L. W., and R. M. Steers. 1973. "Organizational Work and Personal Factors in Employee Turnover and Absenteeism." *Psychological Bulletin* 80 (2):151–76.

Prochaska, J. O., C. C. DiClemente, and J. C. Norcross, J. C. 1992. "In Search of How People Change: Applications to Addictive Behaviors." *American Journal of Psychology*, 47 (9): 1102–14.

Prochaska, J. O., J. C. Norcross, and C. C. DiClemente. 1994. *Changing for Good*. New York: Morrow.

Prochaska, J. O. and W. F. Velicer. 1997. "The Transtheoretical Model of Health Behavior Change." *American Journal of Health Promotion* 12 (1): 38–48.

Satinsky, M. A. 1995 *An Executive Guide to Case Management Strategies*. Chicago: American Hospital Publishers.

Smith, H. L., and M. Fottler. 1998. "Training and Development." In *Essentials of Human Resources Management in Health Services Organizations*, edited by M. Fottler, S. R. Hernandez, and C. L. Joiner. Albany, NY: Delmar Publishers.

PHYSICIAN INVOLVEMENT

To most, a discussion of physician involvement in population health management seems mandatory. As major providers of healthcare, physicians must be involved to manage the health of a population. Nonetheless, as described in many chapters in this book, strategies for population health management do not always revolve around physicians. Demand management strategies may be overseen by physicians, but nurses and nonclinical personnel typically provide the bulk of services. Although physicians often are central in disease management, the focus of many programs may be driven by the concerns of payers or institutions rather than by individual physicians.

For population health to be appropriately and effectively managed, physicians must be involved. Physicians play a central role in the healthcare delivery process and serve as key members of care management teams. Including physicians in the larger picture of managing population health ensures that initiatives accommodate reasonable clinical concerns and maintain a focus on both individual and population health.

This chapter highlights the pivotal role of physicians in all population health management strategies. Hopefully such a consideration will facilitate the inclusion of physicians in population health, which, in turn, will allow programs to succeed in attaining health management and health improvement goals.

Physician Roles

As in general clinical practice, roles for physicians in population health management vary widely. Beyond their role as medical care providers, physicians can serve as patient advocates, patient educators, or program designers. Physicians also play an important role in program communications, coordination, and data collection. They serve crucial roles as experts as they monitor the quality of care and health outcomes, and they can extend all of their roles if they serve as medical directors for population health management programs. In these different roles, physicians can encourage their patients to strive toward better health and help them attain it.

Physician as Clinician

In population health management programs physicians are, of course, direct providers of medical care services. Whether primary care providers or specialists, physicians direct and provide care for their patients. Relying on a combination of training, experience, research, and guidance from program information such as pathways or protocols, physicians deliver medical care to the patients who seek their services. This fundamental role puts physicians in direct contact with patients where they can help to improve individual health and well-being through their treatments. These patient care interactions provide opportunities for physicians to make suggestions about modifying health risks and changing unhealthy behaviors in the interest of improving clinical, functional, and financial outcomes for both patients and payers.

Physician as Patient Advocate

Physician providers often note that they serve as a critical link between the patients they treat and the fiscal intermediary trying to define the level or amount of care that can or should be provided to individual patients. The declining reputation of health maintenance organizations and managed care (Blendon et al. 1998; Wehrwein 1997a) is only one indication of the public's view of the third-party payer as an unnecessary obstructionist limiting well-intentioned providers and hopeful patients in their quest for more and better medical care.

As evidenced by the Hippocratic oath they take before beginning clinical practice, physicians are dedicated to the ideals of doing no harm and helping their patients to the best of their abilities. However, because resources are scarce in healthcare as in other sectors of the economy, physicians are unable to do absolutely everything possible for every patient. Instead, physicians must effectively manage a patient's consumption of healthcare resources within the constraints set forth by the payer.

A physician's role as patient advocate emerges in this environment of constrained resources. While payers place limits on the amount and types of care available for covered individuals, physicians make requests about the best and most appropriate types of medical care for their patients. When such requests are in conflict with the limits ascribed by payers, physicians often advocate on behalf of their patients to emphasize the medical necessity of proposed treatments and care processes.

The ideal of population health management is that by acknowledging existing financial constraints, medical care provision can be more effectively allocated within a defined population. By applying techniques such as demand and disease management, both patients and providers become better informed, thus better able to make good choices about the medical services they demand and use.

Given constrained resources for medical care provision, many steps can be taken by patients, providers, and even employers to encourage individuals to improve consumer health behaviors and reduce their need for costly medical interventions. Then, when prevention efforts deteriorate and medical care is necessary, attention to issues such as efficiency, appropriateness, and cost-effectiveness in the context of health management can extend the range of medical care resources available for a given population.

In this model, physician providers play a critical role as gatekeepers for medical care services. Both by informing their patient consumers and by making care delivery choices consistent with the goals of appropriate use and reasonable allocation of healthcare resources, physicians can serve as advocates for their patients and for the healthcare system.

Physician as Patient Educator

Another vital role for physician providers is that of educators. Although the formal role of health educator may be occupied by nurses or nonclinical health education personnel, the importance of physician involvement in this task is clear. By taking time during clinical appointments to educate patients about their diseases or conditions and making specific recommendations about how to improve health habits and lifestyles, physicians can have a definite effect on patient health. For hypertensive patients, for example, physicians can make suggestions about the importance of losing weight or lowering stress to better manage their disease as well as lower the risk of future health problems from uncontrolled blood pressure. Unfortunately, physician participation in this role as health educators is inconsistent. Physician time is increasingly constrained, and there are few obvious incentives to encourage physicians to take the time necessary to provide health and wellness advice.

Population health management strategies often rely heavily on patient education to accomplish their health improvement goals. Demand management programs, for example, use health education extensively to inform patients about appropriate demand for medical care services and about effective self-care opportunities. Similarly, disease management programs include health education modules to educate individuals about their diseases, including symptoms to monitor, opportunities for self-care, and appropriate times to call a physician. Keeping physicians involved in the oversight of the health education components of population management programs ensures that the educational material provided—whether from literature, the Internet, or individuals providing advice over the telephone—is not contradictory and is consistent with good medical practice.

Physician as Program Designer

Physicians involved in population health management also have the opportunity to participate in such programs by aiding in program design. Whether a program begins as a demand management strategy emphasizing self-care or a disease management strategy reliant upon physician involvement to specify treatment plans, physicians can play a pivotal role if they choose to get involved in program design. The clinical knowledge and practice experience physicians bring to program design is invaluable in developing an effective and appropriate health management program.

For demand management programs, physicians can assist with program design by developing or refining protocols and decision support algorithms to guide patients toward self-care options or direct them to various medical care providers. Disease management programs are dependent upon physician involvement in the development of practice guidelines and care protocols. As an added benefit, getting physicians involved in program design can lead to more effective recruitment of other physicians to participate as providers for patient participants. Catastrophic care management programs provide opportunities for physicians to design program criteria for provider referrals and guidelines for appropriate expected outcomes for patients. Disability management programs can use occupational health providers to devise strategies for injury and illness reduction in the workplace. Physicians interested in disability management can help design protocols to diagnose and treat disabled workers as well as help devise rehabilitation strategies and return-to-work expectations consistent with program goals. Furthermore, physicians can extend their role as participating clinicians by helping to design treatment protocols, defining criteria for modified work, and working with worksite health promotion programs and opportunities.

Physician involvement in program design for population health management is, in fact, mandatory. Physicians offer required clinical insight as well as serving as major players providing and directing appropriate care in different medical settings. Keeping physicians involved at the level of population health management program design can ensure reasonable program activities and attainable program goals.

Physician as Communicator and Coordinator

Probably one of the most important aspects of physician involvement in medical care is communication. Physicians must communicate with patients, family members, other clinicians, administrators, and many others who comprise the teams of individuals concerned and involved in the care of those patients. In the context of population health management, this communication becomes critical when physicians are participating in health management strategies developed to optimize population health. Physicians are responsible for communicating about health promotion and education strategies as well as about appropriate self-care measures. For patients with chronic conditions, physicians must communicate about the best ways for these individuals to manage their diseases. Communications about medications, necessary tests, and provider follow-up must be clearly understood by patients to ensure their compliance with appropriate treatment regimens. When other family members or friends are involved in caring for a patient, these individuals must also be included in physician communications.

Particularly critical is physician communication with other providers. Physicians must be able to communicate with physicians, nurses, and other caregivers across multiple settings. In the context of a population health management program, communications between nurse care managers and physicians must be clear and understood so that patients receive optimal care. Other involved providers must also be included in the communication process to make sure patients do not receive conflicting advice about either self-care or the need to seek medical care.

Coordination among providers is also vital to the success of a population health management strategy. Especially when different programs are involved, coordination between the programs is important to make sure that individual participants are receiving consistent messages about their health management. When programs are supported by information technologies that facilitate such coordination, physicians benefit when they can obtain easy access to this information. However, when information technologies are limited or when physicians do not have access to the data, the coordination challenge is best met by enhanced verbal communications among care providers and program participants.

In any care situation that involves patients switching providers and sites of care, coordination is critical. Patients who are hospitalized and then discharged to a sub-acute care facility or to home for follow-up home healthcare create management challenges for their care teams. Not only are patients receiving care and advice in multiple settings, but frequently the medical records and physician recommendations associated with their treatments do not follow the individual patients. To prevent coordination problems or gaps in overall care management, high-quality population health management programs ensure that coordinators such as care managers (as discussed in Chapter 12) closely monitor their patients and their care needs. The attention and information tracked by these care managers is invaluable to participating physicians who may not be familiar with the treatment progress and recommendations made prior to each physician's encounter with the patient.

For patients with chronic conditions whose management involves multiple providers, coordinating the service provision and recommendations of these providers reduces duplication of services as well as patient confusion. Multiple provider health management programs such as disability management strategies or programs for catastrophic care management become particularly vulnerable to these challenges. Even demand management strategies overseen by physicians have the potential to confuse the individual patient who is under the care of a regular physician if that physician is not familiar with the demand management program.

Ideally, population health management programs should be designed to reduce coordination problems and help participating physicians care for their patients in the most appropriate ways possible. By sharing information among providers and programs, involved physicians can promote consistent health management advice while minimizing coordination problems.

Physician as Information Source

Physicians serve a vital function in population health management when they collect information about their patients. Physicians drive data collection by specifying what data are important to track the clinical and functional health of their patients. While physicians themselves may not serve as data collectors, information about patients' conditions, treatments, medications, status, and so forth is important for health management overall. Programs supported by information technologies may facilitate the role of physicians as data collectors by providing access to appropriate technologies at the point of care. For physicians who can track patients using handheld devices such as personal data assistants (PDAs) or bedside computers, data collection will become second nature and be incorporated into a patient care routine. However, in programs where physicians are reliant upon paper records and order sheets, the data collection role is often delegated to individuals who support the physician, or to care managers involved in the health management program.

Because of the depth of physicians' clinical knowledge as well as their ongoing involvement with individual patients, physician involvement in data collection is crucial. Clinical information must be tracked from visits or telephone consults, medication regimens must be monitored, and health management program coordinators must be aware of necessary patient follow-up recommended by treating physicians. Documentation is clearly important in the medical care environment as a whole; therefore, extending this need for clear and constant collection of information and documentation in a population health management framework is consistent with other required physician activities.

Physician as Expert: Providing Quality and Clinical Oversight

Another critical role for physicians in population health management strategies is to provide the clinical oversight vitally needed for any medical program. Because such programs necessarily involve discussing and working with health and medical care issues, physician providers are often the most highly trained program participants. The extensive training and experience of most involved physicians can ensure that program recommendations are appropriate, consistent, and logical. Having physicians involved in such programs from the outset can improve overall program quality (Golembesky 1999). By overseeing health management guidelines and protocols with an eye towards ultimate program goals such as improved health and better clinical outcomes, physician providers offer the depth and breadth of oversight necessary for program success.

Guidelines and protocols must be developed and/or approved by physicians who will provide the care recommended in such cases. In the case of most population health management strategies, various protocols, care maps, and decision support aids are designed based on an underlying clinical logic that must be developed and approved by physicians. Demand management care pathways specifying when patients can appropriately care for themselves and when they need to be seen by a physician must be reviewed by physicians. Similarly, the advice provided over the phone by nurse care managers, social workers, or disease management counselors should be coordinated with clinical goals established by physicians. In the case of disability management programs, both the determination of disability and appropriate expectations for rehabilitation and clinical progress must be guided by physicians. Ongoing professional oversight is mandatory in the context of population health management programs where the primary concern is patient health.

In addition to clinical program oversight, physicians should also serve an important role in peer review. Most population health management strategies are developed with a necessary focus on desired outcomes and goals for the programs. Because many of the activities incorporated in population health management involve clinicians, such activities are subject to review. Programs that track outcomes by individual provider offer opportunities for peer comparison and formal peer review. While all patients are admittedly unique, physicians whose treatment patterns regularly fall outside program performance norms may be identifiable and can be considered for more intensive professional review. Individual physicians can help with this peer review process as well as monitor stated program goals for their appropriateness. These types of activities support the physician role in quality and oversight, ensuring that program strategies are suitable and that provider behaviors are consistent with program goals.

Physician as Innovator: Integration of Alternative and Complementary Medicine

Physicians who are knowledgeable of, and open to, complementary and alternative medicine (CAM) also play an important role in population health management strategies. CAM is increasing in popularity in the United States, and evidence of its effectiveness is growing. Physicians open to the possibilities of working with CAM providers or strategies can be very valuable within a population health management strategy that includes such options. Whether their role is for referral to CAM providers, serving as a physician provider of CAM, or merely coordinating treatment regimens between traditional and CAM options, physicians can make a difference in the health and well-being of their patients.

Physician as Medical Director

A different role that physicians play in population health management is that of medical directors. Large programs often have a medical director employed either full-time or part-time for the benefit of their participants. However, even smaller programs and those that are outsourced to contracted vendors typically retain some sort of formal medical direction by a physician provider.

Whether serving as official program directors or as in-house medical directors for institutions where population health management programs are in place, this oversight role is very important. Physician medical directors may retain clinical responsibilities or may serve as full-time medical directors with all of their time devoted to managerial and programmatic concerns. Depending on physicians' interests, this role can be very appealing. Physicians interested in both the management and policy sides of medical care will enjoy the opportunity to have influence in both areas by serving in this medical director role.

Physician Involvement in Different Population Health Management Programs

Each of the different population health management strategies discussed in this book relies on physician involvement to a greater or lesser degree. Lifestyle and demand management strategies may depend less on direct physician involvement but require the support and oversight of physicians to ensure proper focus on health behaviors and health and care management opportunities. Disease and catastrophic care management programs depend on constant physician involvement to provide clinical care and case oversight, while disability management programs can use physicians peripherally or centrally, depending on program focus and goals.

Disease and catastrophic care management programs both rely heavily on physician involvement to deliver care to program participants. Disease management programs are typically designed to give physicians specific clinical guidance about managing a particular disease within the context of the program. Parameters such as frequency of visits, clinical and functional outcomes to be monitored, or drug therapies to be considered are often specified in a disease management program. Optimally, specification of these parameters can standardize care for program patients and improve disease and cost outcomes for the patient and payer. Catastrophic care management programs have a similar clinical component and may also include parameters designed to facilitate coordination of multiple physician specialists to manage and optimize care for catastrophically ill and injured individuals.

Demand and lifestyle management programs usually operate with less constant physician involvement, yet physician acceptance of these strategies for population health management is key to program success. Involvement of physicians in the design and development of these health management strategies improves the likelihood of program success by ensuring adequate attention to clinical concerns and evidence for health behavior change opportunities. Without physician oversight of a clinically based program, provider institutions are less likely to accept and recommend use of demand management services. Sound demand management programs that use telephone advice, apply nurse-led protocols, or provide information about health and wellness to inbound callers rely upon physicians to approve triage protocols and sources of health education information. Further, commercial demand management companies rely upon consistent and committed physician involvement in their programs to validate their approach to population health management and improvement. Including physicians in these programs ensures quality of care and facilitates better attainment of health improvement goals.

Involvement of physicians in disability management programs is also crucial. Primary care physicians and specialists must be informed about requirements and legal issues surrounding disability cases. The need to coordinate both employee and employer awareness about the nature and progress of disease and disability requires substantial understanding and involvement on the part of physician providers. Programs focusing on risk reduction and injury prevention benefit from clinical oversight by knowledgeable occupational health specialists. Furthermore, when employees do become disabled, dedicated physician providers concerned about improving care and health for the defined population of employees served can be very important members of multidisciplinary care teams.

Physician Resistance

Involvement of physicians in population health management programs, while vital, often proves difficult. Physician resistance takes many forms ranging from discomfort with population health management overall to concern that a specific program will not be flexible enough to respond to the needs of individual patients. Many physicians feel they already provide health and care management services under the heading of "patient management" (Wehrwein 1997b) as they provide ongoing care services to their patients. Some view disease management programs as "cookbook medicine" that threatens to take the "art" out of medical practice. Trained to be independent, physicians may be uncomfortable using the team-based models of most population health management strategies. Similarly, program outreach and long-distance monitoring may not be skills physicians have developed in their practices (Wynn 1996).

Physicians are often barraged by a large number of different program requirements with varied practice guidelines, many of which are contradictory, and most of which change on a regular basis ("Physician" 1998). Understandably, physicians become resentful when they perceive that programs are thinly veiled cost-containment strategies attempting to enforce physician compliance with financially based protocols. Requirements to incorporate new information technology, if expensive or unreasonable, create additional sources of physician resistance (Terry 1998a; 1998b). Furthermore, the time required for program activities such as patient education and data collection from one or multiple programs can be overwhelming, unrealistic, and unreimbursed ("Physician" 1998).

Overcoming physician resistance to program participation is mandatory. Harry Leider (2001) has presented a list of tactics that he considers key to achieving physician buy-in, including:

- providing physician education;
- enlisting physician champions;
- building on demonstrated program success;
- sharing program gains; and
- giving physicians tools to participate.

Providing physician education involves reassuring physicians that they will be able to maintain professional autonomy and their central role as patient care providers in the program. Providing evidence of favorable program outcomes that demonstrate the value of adding population health management tactics such as patient education, monitoring of patient compliance, and other care management tools can also be very effective (Leider 2001).

Enlisting physician champions encourages visible support from physician opinion leaders in the local community. One programmatic approach to encourage physician participation uses advisory boards or physician advisory committees of specialists and primary care physicians to support the population health management program. Advisory board members can be educated about population health management concepts and practices while they are consulted for their views about program development and implementation. Physicians can provide valuable input to many decisions including building versus outsourcing a program, selecting vendors, modifying clinical guidelines, identifying patients, and implementing the program in practice (Leider 2001). Many programs have also found that involving physicians in program design makes the program more attractive and acceptable to those physicians who would be appropriate participants.

Building on program success describes the importance of demonstrating to physicians that population health management techniques succeed in practice. When implementing a disease management program, for example, one strategy for success is to initially target diseases for which favorable and timely outcomes are fairly easy to achieve. Instead of focusing on low back pain or osteoporosis, programs that start with asthma or congestive heart failure may be easier to implement and demonstrate good results. Diseases associated with comorbidities such as diabetes and programs with misaligned financial incentives are typically more difficult to implement (Leider 2001) and can be included later as program success grows and providers demonstrate commitment.

Sharing program gains with physicians involves providing financial incentives, when feasible, to spark physician interest in participation. If possible, providing population health management fees to compensate physicians for their time can be very effective. Incentive structures such as bonus programs or pay for performance can also be intriguing. Provision of physician stipends for their roles in program design or program management are also considered reasonable approaches to sharing program gains (Leider 2001).

Programs should also reflect the absolute necessity of *giving physicians tools* to manage their individual patients and patient populations more effectively. Clear reports, efficient interactions with care managers, and judicious presentation of data from remote care monitoring situations all support physicians as they treat and manage their patients (Leider 2001). Evidence has shown that physicians will typically work with population health management programs if the initiative helps reduce their workload and can demonstrate improvement in patient health and in the quality of care provided to their patients (Ritterband 2000). As an example, organizations can monitor how patients enrolled in a specific disease management program are being treated, and lists of patients who need follow-up appointments or certain tests can be provided to physicians to assist them in their practice (Cross 1998). This type of feedback improves both quality of care and service to patients.

Ideally, population health management strategies can be developed to improve and coordinate care for people in multiple ways that support the work of physicians. Instead of intending to reduce the amount of care provided by physicians, programs should assist primary care physicians in treating their patients in the most appropriate and efficient ways. The limited time available for education and extended discussion in physician office visits can be supplemented by components of disease management programs, for example, that emphasize health education and clinical support by nonphysician providers such as nurse case managers and nurse educators (Wynn 1996; Terry 1998a). These additional medical personnel can be charged with taking care of their patients enrolled in different programs, making sure that the patients' physicians are alerted when clinical conditions change or show a need for physician involvement. Similarly, population health management programs can educate their involved physicians about the processes of care they are managing (Isham 1997), helping physicians to provide and coordinate better quality of care for their patients. Attempting to make physicians' lives easier with the tools and services of population health management can reduce physician resistance to participation and improve the quality of care and service for the program.

Delivering Patient-Centered Care

Delivering appropriate care focused on the needs of individual patients represents another important role for physicians in population health management. The traditional medical care system has been largely focused on diseases or organ systems, centering action upon acute events. Population health management strategies provide an opportunity to personalize healthcare and make the system more patient-centric (Wehrwein 1997) when care is delivered. While the recent push in medicine is toward standardization, reduction of variation, and increased application of evidence-based medicine, it is the critical role of the physician to respond to the specific needs and circumstances of individual patients. Regardless of the health characteristics and epidemiology of the defined population served, individual patients are treated by individual physicians who must be responsive to their individual needs.

The allure of evidence-based medicine is that it can provide clinical guidance for physicians struggling to determine the best way to care for patients. Rather than relying on anecdotal experiences, evidence-based medicine can help organize and synthesize the clinical and scientific evidence available about particular conditions and treatments. However, evidence-based medicine relies on the premise that statistical analyses of groups of individuals can prescribe the one best way to care for individual patients. This logic may be inherently flawed when an individual physician is confronted with a single patient. Instead of relying on results obtained from the aggregate data analyzed in the evidence gathering process, the physician must cull relevant information and apply it to the individual sitting in his or her office (Tanenbaum 1993). As Sandra Tanenbaum (1994) notes, much of physician reasoning is deterministic, and physicians rely heavily on knowledge gained from personal experience. Participation in different programs builds a foundation of physician knowledge and experience based on providing care and service in the context of population health management. Further, when programs are supported by information technologies that permit modification of protocols and algorithms based upon knowledge gained about individual patient perceptions and circumstances, physicians can use this information to deliver personalized and appropriate patient-centered care.

Delivering patient-centered care is consistent with the business concept of mass customization, which relies on the assumption that it is possible to define both market and business relationships in a way that is specific and unique for each customer (Coile 1998). The notion of mass customization has emerged around the development of technologies that make it possible to provide consumers with products or services that are standardized but delivered in a way that is customized to fit the needs of the individual consumer (Davis 1996). As the knowledge base and expectations of healthcare consumers increase, these customers demand personalized attention and medical care that is appropriate and effective. Innovations such as the Internet, information networks, integrated databases, artificial intelligence, and expert systems facilitate this customization process. For example, examination rooms equipped with Internet access enable the physician and patient to work together to search for current and appropriate disease and health education information (Engstrom 1997).

Delivering patient-centered care is crucial for population health management programs that attempt to improve the health and well-being of a population by intervening with individuals. Patients need help from physicians and other providers to make better decisions about both their health behaviors and their need to seek medical care (Paul 2000). A population health management strategy can be developed based on system capabilities to obtain, analyze, and synthesize data from multiple sources. With defined populations to serve, these programs provide natural settings to apply tools such as clinical guidelines, pathways, and care plans. Evaluation of data for these populations permits assessment of health risks and identification of individuals who are predicted to be high-risk. Because such identification is possible, health and care management plans can be customized to the needs of those high-risk individuals to reduce their risk levels, thus better managing resources available to the population as a whole.

Information Technology

Physician use of information and information technologies presents another important challenge in population health management. When population health management strategies rely upon data to select or intervene on individual patients, those data must accurately reflect patient conditions. Physicians, as primary members of patient care teams, often determine the data elements upon which care decisions are based. Information such as diagnosis codes or medications originate from physicians assessing patients and prescribing treatment regimens. Not only are physicians initially responsible for the data upon which risk assessments and case-mix adjustments are based, but physicians must use the results of such evaluations as they care for patients on an ongoing basis. Timeliness and accuracy of data must be ensured to facilitate appropriate and informed clinical decisions that are aided by access to such information.

The use and integration of data become more complicated as various information technologies are introduced in clinical practice. As more and more information comes closer to the patient bedside or provider office, physicians play an increasingly important role in translating clinical data into patient care practices. Evidence suggests that computer-based clinical decision support tools can improve physician performance, especially in the areas of determining drug dosage, providing preventive care reminders, and quality assurance (Johnston et al. 1994). Treatment guidelines or medication lists available on a PDA or a bedside terminal provide guidance to physicians in a variety of situations. However, practicing physicians must be able to interpret suggested treatment guidelines and to evaluate if the care prescribed is indeed appropriate for the patient sitting in front of them.

This assessment must proceed more and more quickly as information technologies enable physicians to access guidelines and treatment information in real time. Physicians must be able to apply these information technologies and care tools while maintaining their own individual perspectives about the patients they see and the circumstances these patients describe. This interpretive process becomes more important as information technologies spread and their use becomes expected in most clinical settings.

Education of Health Professionals

A final consideration for physicians involved in and committed to population health management is the education of physicians and other health professionals. Deciding to adopt a population health management strategy that takes into consideration the needs and health of a defined population has implications for the future of healthcare education. Medical schools are already stretched to expose students to the comprehensive body of medical knowledge and skills required for individuals to become doctors. However, the development of new models of clinical practice and care management will provide more challenges for new physicians.

Opportunities exist in medical education to consider a population perspective. Courses in epidemiology and biostatistics introduce students to the concepts of population health and analysis. Strategies for population health management are not inconsistent with medical training, but the notion of managing health for a population of patients rather than only the individuals themselves is often a different concept for new physicians. Instead of focusing on individuals, population health management strategies try to allocate health resources in ways that will offer the most impact for the population as a whole. For instance, if an elderly population is targeted, influenza immunizations may be an emphasis for the members of that demographic group. For the individual physician provider with a panel of patients of different ages, this focus may be either welcome or annoying, especially when extra record-keeping is required. Depending on how interventions are promoted for individuals within the managed population, physicians will either feel comfortable with such programs or at constant odds with treatment recommendations. Physicians who choose to practice in managed care settings will be familiar with the concept of financial risk by necessity, but physicians who are newly exposed to the financial management aspects of health management strategies may be uncomfortable with the parameters of these programs.

From an individual patient perspective, population health management strategies try to leverage the tools of information technology, data analysis, and risk screening to identify specific individuals who will benefit from targeted interventions. In practice, the interventions offered through programs such as disease or disability management should not be contradictory to standard clinical practice. However, the notion that such patients are being continually monitored throughout the medical care system may create challenges for physicians in coordination, communication, and data management.

Not all physicians are familiar with the tools of population health management as described in this text. Although survey methodology and risk screening are often appropriately delegated to health services researchers with expertise in these areas, physician involvement in the interpretation of such information in clinical practice is critical. Similarly, designing behavioral interventions or program evaluations may not be projects appropriate for all physicians. Instead, the opportunity for clinicians may be to participate, to the extent possible and desired, in determining treatment options and care pathways appropriate for health management programs. Even though physicians may not have experience developing guidelines or care protocols, this fundamental program task can only be done with the involvement of clinicians.

Ideally, multidisciplinary teams of clinicians, researchers, and managers can work together to design and implement such pathways for health management programs. Clinician involvement is mandatory to ensure that such guidelines include not only proper treatments, but information about cases that would be exceptions in treatment guidelines. Practicing physicians must also keep the reasonableness of guidelines and protocols in mind as they provide care for individual patients. Although this type of reasoned clinical logic is well supported by medical education, applying such techniques in a population health management approach is still somewhat new.

Conclusion

Physicians involved in population health management must consider the multiple potential roles they play. Their role as patient advocates helps them keep their patients' best interests in mind as they provide individualized treatment within a population health management framework. The importance of physicians' roles as communicators is also clear. They serve another important function in program coordination as they help coordinate patient care, work with information technology, and even facilitate program data collection.

Beyond their communication and coordination roles, physicians in any health management program are both clinicians and experts. Physicians practicing clinical medicine serve a special role for patients and program developers as they perform program interventions within the guidelines of good medical care. In practice, the physician role as expert in medicine cannot be underemphasized. As practicing physicians or medical directors, physicians have received medical training that sets them aside as experts in health and healthcare. This expertise gives them an important opportunity to design appropriate programs, interventions, and treatments in the context of health improvement for any population.

Whether serving as a program medical director, clinical advisor, or participating provider, physician involvement in population health management strategies benefits both patients and the programs themselves. Population health management programs can be designed to support and enhance patients' relationships with their physician providers, and physician satisfaction can increase with the support of a well-run population health management program that is consistent with clinical practice and patient care goals. The combined efforts of program personnel and involved physician providers produce high-quality care and program activities that enable population health management programs to succeed.

REFERENCES

Blendon, R. J., M. Brodie, J. M. Benson, D. E. Altman, L. Levitt, T. Hoff, and L. Hugick. 1998. "Understanding the Managed Care Backlash." *Health Affairs* 17 (4): 80–94.

Coile, R. C. 1998. *Millenium Management*. Chicago: Health Administration Press.

Cross, M. 1998. "Needed: Strategies to Get Physicians to 'Buy in' to Disease Management." *Managed Care* (May). [On-line article; retrieved 2/5/01.] http://www.managedcaremag.com/archives/9805/9805. buyin.shtml.

Davis, S. 1996. *Future Perfect*. Reading, MA: Addison-Wesley Publishing Company.

Engstrom, P. 1997. "Net-linked Exam Rooms Open Up New Vistas for Both MDs and Patients." *Medicine on the Net* 3 (2): 1–2.

Golembesky, H. E. 1999. "Developing Disease Management Programs." *Healthcare Executive* 14 (5): 39–40.

Isham, G. 1997. "Population Health and HMOs: The Partners for Better Health Experience." *Healthcare Forum Journal* 40 (6): 36–39.

Johnston, M. E., K. B. Langton, R. B. Haynes, and A. Mathieu. 1994. "Effects of Computer-based Clinical Decision Support Systems on Clinician Performance and Patient Outcome." *Annals of Internal Medicine* 120 (2): 135–42.

Leider, H. 2001. "Gaining Physician Buy-in—The "Achilles Heel" of Disease Management." *E-CareManagement News* (May 2). [On-line article; retrieved 1/20/02.] http://bhtinfo.com/05_02_01.htm.

Paul, K. A. 2000. "Managing the Demand for Health Services by Adopting Patient-centered Programs." *Benefits Quarterly* (Second Quarter): 54–59.

"Physician Buy-in to DM Programs Becomes Big Hurdle." 1998. *Disease Management News* (July 25). [On-line article; retrieved 3/3/02.] http://www.phdx.com/corporate/corporate_resource_doc.html.

Ritterband, D. R. 2000. "Disease Management: Old Wine in New Bottles?" *Journal of Healthcare Management* 45 (4): 255–66.

Tanenbaum, S. J. 1993. "What Physicians Know." *New England Journal of Medicine* 329 (17): 1268–71.

Tanenbaum, S. J. 1994. "Knowing and Acting in Medical Practice: The Epistemological Politics of outcomes Research." *Journal of Health Politics, Policy and Law* 19 (1): 27–44.

Terry, K. 1998a."The Disease-Management Boom: How Doctors Are Dealing With It." *Medical Economics* (April 27): 60–72.

Terry, K. 1998b. "Here's What's Coming—Like It or Not." *Medical Economics* 1998 (April 27): 72–99.

Wehrwein, P. 1997a. "Why Managed Care Is Getting a Bad Rap." *Managed Care* (February). [On-line article; retrieved 6/4/02.] http://www.managedcaremag.com/archiveMC/9702/9702.badrap.shtml.

Wehrwein, P. 1997b. "Disease Management Gains a Degree of Respectability." *Managed Care* (August). [On-line article; retrieved 6/4/02.] http://www.managedcaremag.com/archiveMC/9708/9708.mainstream.html.

Wynn, P. 1996. "The Role of Physicians in Disease Management." *Managed Care* (October). [On-line article; retrieved 6/4/02.] http://www.managedcaremag.com/archives/9610/MC9610.diseasemgmt.shtml.

INFORMATION TECHNOLOGY

Information technology (IT) is a critical component of effective and efficient population health management. From preliminary health assessments to final outcomes analyses, IT facilitates the health management process. Computers maintain databases of potential participants, facsimile machines improve coordination and understanding among providers and program staff, and increasingly sophisticated telephonic devices promote communications in a variety of ways.

However, despite rapid innovation in business information technologies, most observers believe that the adoption of IT in healthcare has been relatively slow. While banks and other financial institutions spend an average of 6.3 percent of revenues on information technologies, healthcare organizations typically spend only 2.2 percent of revenues on IT (itmWEB 2002). Calculating IT investment per employee, other industries such as banking and insurance spend nearly five times the amount spent in the healthcare industry. Instead, many healthcare processes rely on paper-based medical records, clinical notes and orders written by hand, and large reference textbooks sitting on office shelves.

Adopting information technologies in a population health management context can be very valuable. Benefits of expanded use of IT include better clinical decision making, increased productivity, improvements in quality of care, reductions in medication errors, streamlined operations, and increased satisfaction for physicians, patients, and employees. As shown in Table 14.1, information is imperative to help population health management strategies achieve their goals. Taking advantage of available and appropriate information technologies can leverage the value and effect of population health management programs as they improve health and well-being for their target populations.

Role of Information Systems and Information Technology

Information systems provide the backbone for many population health management strategies. Data collection, organization, and analysis are facilitated by information systems, and remote care management and monitoring extend the reach and impact of different population health management programs. Information technologies also play an important role as decision support tools. Automation of patient care guidelines, pathways, and health

TABLE 14.1
Population
Health
Management
Goals and
Information
Imperatives

Population Health Management Goals	Information Imperatives
Focus on wellness, disease prevention, care management of defined populations	• Population profiles, epidemiology • Individual propensity for disease • Medical and nonmedical prevention
Systematic implementation of clinical guidelines, protocols, care pathways	• Clinical decision criteria • Variation from current guidelines • Guideline effectiveness and improvement opportunities
Seamless provision of care across multiple settings and multiple providers	• Intervention history tracked by location • Care plans and actions taken recorded • Capabilities of each setting known
Member and family participation in care planning and decision making	• Family relationships • Access to information about self-diagnosis, self-care, and self-management
Establishing outcome targets and parameters	• Stratified outcomes (disability, quality of life, functional status, social factors) • Total care history • Cost
Emergence of virtual organizations of providers, suppliers, and purchasers	• Risk-sharing arrangements by entity • Revenues and costs attributed to each entity • Resource availability by organization

SOURCE: Adapted from: Moore, G. B., B. E. Reynolds, and D. A. Ray. 1995. "Information Architects: Data by Design." *HMO Magazine* 36 (3): 29–31, 34–35.

assessments can improve both the quality and effectiveness of population health management strategies. Figure 14.1 illustrates some of the many benefits of including information technologies in population health management strategies. Furthermore, Table 14.2 provides examples of how information technologies can be applied in different population health management programs.

Data Collection, Organization, and Analysis

Information systems are of obvious importance in the design, development, and implementation of population health management programs. First, to define a population to manage, it is important that data be available by which to identify target participants. Potential participants are usually screened by evaluating existing data sources such as those containing demographic, clinical, pharmacological, and financial information. A review of

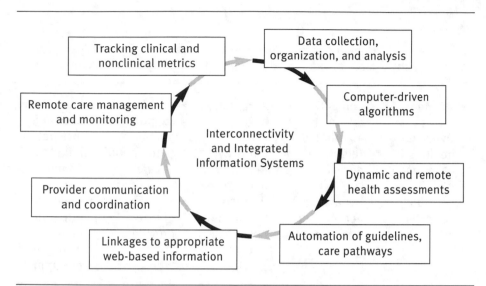

FIGURE 14.1
Information
Technology
Facilitates
Population
Health
Management

SOURCE: McAlearney, A. S. 2002. "Population Health Management in Theory and Practice." In *Advances in Health Care Management* (Volume 3), edited by G. T. Savage, J. Blair, and M. Fottler. New York: JAI Press/Elsevier Science Ltd.

hospital claims, outpatient visits, health plan surveys, employee databases, health risk assessments, pharmacy claims, and other data sources will identify individual members of defined populations who can be targeted for population health management interventions. Programs that rely mainly on analysis of administrative claims data may suffer because of both the quality and timeliness of the data available. The ability to combine multiple sources of data to describe and define a population facilitates appropriate targeting and tailoring of program activities.

Organization of data is also important. Programs that do not have sophisticated information systems capabilities will have problems maintaining ongoing enrollment in a program if they cannot quickly and accurately identify appropriate participants. In contrast, organizations with access to appropriate information systems can apply criteria by which to screen patients and members for participation in a population health management program and can maintain a continuous flow of appropriate patients into the program. Integration of databases and information systems facilitates both the targeting and health and care management processes necessary to support an ongoing program.

Other important aspects of information systems capabilities are the abilities to analyze various data and to measure outcomes. Population health management programs that establish goals and objectives up front must be able to both capture baseline measurements and evaluate program outcomes in light of those goals. Beyond simple counts, the ability to analyze program data to measure program progress and effects is very important. Furthermore, the extent to which data collection and analysis can be

TABLE 14.2
Information
Technology
Applications
in Population
Health
Management

Lifestyle Management	Demand Management	Disease Management	Catastrophic Care Management	Disability Management
• Tailored messages • Dynamic health assessments • Web-based self-care education	• Computer-driven algorithms • Telephonic decision support • Dynamic health assessments	• Automation of guidelines, care pathways • Remote care management/ disease monitoring • Coordination of care providers	• Web-based support groups • Automation of care guidelines • Coordination of care providers	• Coordination of benefits • Integrated benefits administration • Ability to integrate absence management programs

SOURCE: McAlearney, A. S. 2002. "Population Health Management in Theory and Practice." In *Advances in Health Care Management* (Volume 3), edited by G. T. Savage, J. Blair, and M. Fottler. New York: JAI Press/Elsevier Science Ltd.

automated can reduce implementation problems and help leverage program resources to address other issues.

Remote Care Management and Monitoring

Remote monitoring of clinical conditions provides another opportunity for information systems and information technologies to help patients and providers in the population health management process. Using telephone-based and computer-monitoring devices, patients can stay connected to their providers and health plans with periodic checks. Furthermore, participant progress can be monitored through telephone contacts, provider visits, and delivery of health education.

Remote monitoring devices enable providers to track issues such as medication compliance and clinical course without using more costly home health visits or calls to participants. Patients with chronic conditions or who have been discharged from the hospital to home for follow-up care may be candidates for remote telemonitoring services. Specifically, information technologies such as electronic scales and blood pressure cuffs permit ongoing review of clinical data. When patients consistently use these devices, remote monitoring can aid in the early detection of potential problems and complications ("Predict" 1998). A disease management program for congestive heart failure, for example, can incorporate electronic scales to transmit patient weights instantaneously to program information systems. When this information indicates a problem, clinical data will be transmitted to medical personnel immediately via pager or another electronic messaging system. By linking patients to telemonitoring systems that record vital signs and clinical status, these information technology tools help providers monitor and react to patient data on an ongoing basis.

Given the prevalence of chronic conditions in America, interest in how to provide timely, cost-effective, and high-quality care is sparking considerable innovation. Various remote patient monitoring devices and companies are emerging in this rapidly expanding industry. As of February 2002, at least 55 companies were identified by Better Health Technologies as "remote patient monitoring" companies providing services or products including medical monitoring, medical devices, telemedicine, disease/condition management, fitness/wellness, sensors, and even smart houses. (For more information, go to www.bhtinfo.com/caremgmt.htm.). Although the demonstrated value of remote patient monitoring remains to be proved definitively, evidence indicates that consumers are adopting these applications and are intrigued by the promise of such devices to improve health and quality of life, increase clinical quality of care, and offer additional peace of mind.

In most cases, reimbursement for devices and services has not been worked out, and issues surrounding privacy, confidentiality, and physician resistance remain. However, the potential to reduce medical errors, improve communication between providers and patients, reduce costs, and improve health are all compelling reasons to consider including remote patient monitoring in population health management strategies.

Decision Support Tools

Information technologies and information systems play as an important a role in population health management as decision support tools. Computer-driven algorithms permit the automation of patient care decision rules to decrease variability in patient care and reduce the likelihood of medical errors. Clinical and care decisions can also be supported by applying information technologies to health assessments and patient identification.

Health surveys and health assessments clearly benefit from the incorporation of information technologies. By translating paper-based surveys into computerized tools that incorporate branching logic, the health assessment process can be automated for both data collection and analysis. Assessments created to take advantage of newer computer technologies and Internet programming techniques become dynamic and can be customized for the individual patient. Instead of having a care manager or patient attempt to skip questions in a pre-set pattern, questions that take into account previous responses can appear on a screen or be asked over the telephone. For example, if a person provides an affirmative answer about having diabetes, a diabetes assessment module can be incorporated into this person's ongoing health assessment in a way that is transparent to the respondent. Development of this dynamic assessment capability can improve both the accuracy of information collected and the quality of care and service provided (Nash 2000).

Computer logic also assists in selecting patients for health management opportunities. Decision rules can be established based on targets for a population health management program such as presence of a disease, risk status, or occurrence of a medical event. Available data can be searched using computer-based algorithms that consider multiple patient selection criteria. In a simple example, health assessment information is combined with claims data to identify individuals at high risk for expensive future medical events. However, more sophisticated searches can leverage the value of integrated information systems by relying on multiple data sources. For instance, identification of individuals with particular diseases proceeds based upon multiple algorithms specifying rules for information obtained from claims, pharmacy data, laboratory data, health assessments, or physician referrals. By integrating information from such dispersed sources, algorithms can be designed that are more or less inclusive, depending on the goals of a health management program.

Protocols and guidelines provide another opportunity to apply computer-driven algorithms in patient care. Automating these algorithms and making them available to care managers or physicians at the bedside or in an office makes such guidelines usable at the point of care. Instead of relying on providers to sift through binders of guidelines and protocols that must specify every contingency and relevant alternative for different possible patient types, automated guidelines sort through the relevant decision rules for the patient that is presented. Decisions about patient care must still be made by the attending physician or care manager, but the range of options to be considered can be narrowed to a reasonable and appropriate list. Rather than deluge providers with all the possible benefits and risks of every decision, the ability to describe patient characteristics such as demographics and prior care experiences can help to refine relevant probabilities and assist clinical decision making.

Implementation of automated guidelines can improve population health management by reducing inappropriate variability in medical practice. When these guidelines are accessible and relevant, decision rules can help make the patient care processes more consistent and thorough. Furthermore, patients benefit by receiving appropriate, high-quality medical care based on available clinical evidence, whenever possible. By moving from paper-based systems to automated patient care guidelines and pathways, more consistent and appropriate use of these decision support aids is facilitated. (See 14.1 "Decision Support Tools" at www.ache.org/pubs/mcalearney/start.cfm.)

Integrated Information Systems

The importance of integrating data from multiple sources and the ability to analyze such data from different perspectives has been emphasized in many instances in this book. In practice, information technologies can have considerably greater reach and power when information systems are integrated or interconnected between systems and sites (Reese and Majzun 2000). To the extent information systems are integrated, the data that can be extracted from such systems becomes even more useful because it tends to be more complete. When clinical systems can combine multiple sources of clinical and administrative data such as medical care data, financial information, pharmacy data, and laboratory information, disease management programs can use these multiple data sources to better target, monitor, and measure patients and their outcomes. The ability to access systems at the same time also permits the design of more complex programming logic and algorithms. These algorithms can be developed to respond to the individual needs and conditions of participant respondents in an approach consistent with the concept of mass customization (Davis 1996) (previously described in Chapter 13) as interventions are delivered to individual patients.

Monitoring participants in health management programs relies heavily upon data and IT. In the absence of automated or integrated information systems, monitoring may progress by means of paper records to track telephone contacts, provider visits, and so forth; however, the likelihood of being able to capitalize on opportunities for participant intervention diminishes considerably. Without automation or integration, it is very difficult to systematize the data analysis and monitoring processes that must proceed over the course of individuals' participation in a health management program. Furthermore, the coordination and communication function emphasized as a critical component of all population health management approaches remains extremely difficult.

As described in the discussion of computer-driven algorithms, their power is increased when multiple information systems are accessible at one time. Not only can more complex algorithms be developed, but the ability of health management programs to more appropriately identify and monitor participants is also enhanced. Once developed, the implementation of such algorithms is made possible with integrated and sophisticated information systems. Such processes can be automated to enhance their reliability and reach for potential program participants.

Outcomes assessment also depends on good data collection and information systems capabilities. Without integration of existing databases, simple outcomes such as counts of visits or telephone calls may still be measured, but the accuracy of such data is often suspect. Sophisticated analyses of multivariate outcomes such as cost-effectiveness simply are not feasible without computerized databases.

Furthermore, by integrating information from multiple information systems, different data sources can be combined with clinical measures to monitor new program outcomes. For example, combining clinical information with financial information permits evaluation of program cost-effectiveness.

For a diabetes disease management program, combined outcomes such as cost per deciliter reduction in hemoglobin A1c can be monitored to both assess program cost-effectiveness and program success. In another example, cost data can be combined with quality of life information, such as that captured in a SF-36 health assessment, to track cost per level of improvement. Depending on the outcomes relevant for the specific program, these combined metrics enable program evaluators to assess program benefits and costs in a different light and provide new information about the program.

The integration of information systems also permits enhanced monitoring of healthcare quality. Rather than rely on process metrics such as waiting times for service or number of rings before telephones are answered, quality can be defined in terms of measures both clinically and personally relevant to participants. Improvements in activities of daily living because of a catastrophic health management program can be tracked and associated with the costs involved, patient satisfaction, family perspectives, and time required. Merely reducing the cost of care for a group of patients can be defined as an insufficient outcome if the true goals of a health management program are to improve patient health and well-being.

Combining the information from multiple databases allows both participants and providers to gain from the potential of health management programs. Outcomes can be defined and agreed on from the perspectives of different observers and program sponsors, and then progress towards such outcomes can be monitored. When patient progress is deemed insufficient, interventions can be initiated to respond to observed problems. Using integrated information for the purposes of population health management increases the likelihood that programs will reach the most appropriate individuals and that they will be modified as necessary, given ongoing information about participants' health status and medical events.

Applying Innovations in Information Technology

The diversity of information technologies applicable in a population health management environment is impressive. Because the information technology environment is extremely dynamic, new technologies and devices appear regularly that hold the potential to improve the performance and capabilities of population health management programs. Therefore, it is important, although often difficult, to make sense of what is available in the information technology market that might be appropriate for the population defined for management. Telemedicine, handheld devices, and technology-assisted drug delivery devices provide three examples of how IT innovations can enhance population health management.

Telemedicine

One IT approach that is increasingly important for population health management is telemedicine. Although not new, the field of telemedicine has been expanding rapidly in recent years. Telemedicine is typically defined as telecommunications and information technologies combined to provide remote medical care. Specifically, telemedicine describes the processes of the transfer of medical data over telephone, facsimile, or video conference. It involves activities ranging from telephonic assessments to network transmissions of radiographs or other diagnostic images, to the complicated technologies of telesurgery (Perednia and Allen 1995; Grigsby et al. 1995; Grigsby and Sanders 1998).

Many current examples of the use of telemedicine exist in population health management. Clinical and health services researchers typically use telephonic surveys as a way to follow up with nonrespondents to mailed surveys. Similarly, telephone follow-up as part of research studies is common, enabling periodic assessment and monitoring of patients' conditions and attitudes regarding their experiences with the healthcare system (Chande et al. 1996; Burstein et al. 1996). Telephonic assessments are also used to collect outcome data about patients, or additional information to permit evaluation of program effectiveness (Derlet et al. 1995; McGrory 1997; Simon et al. 1997).

Another common use of telemedicine is to perform healthcare interventions via the telephone. Programs such as smoking cessation initiatives (Rolnick et al. 1997), programs to promote preventive health (Marcus and Crane 1998), and telephone follow-up to provide education and reinforce compliance behaviors for individuals with chronic diseases (Patton et al. 1997) have proved to be acceptable and effective. These techniques can be used in any or all of the five population health management strategies previously described.

Distance technology applications such as computerized communication, telephone follow-up and counseling, telephone reminders, interactive telephone systems, after-hours telephone access, and telephone screening have demonstrated their general effectiveness, especially in the areas of preventive care, management of osteoarthritis, cardiac rehabilitation, and diabetes care (Balas et al. 1997). Benefits from these distance technologies include improved access and support for coordination of clinician activities, enhanced communication between clinicians and patients, and among clinicians. Again, these applications have obvious value in each of the population health management strategies described in this text. (See 14.2 "Telemedicine Programs" at www.ache.org/pubs/mcalearney/ start.cfm.)

Finally, telemedicine approaches can improve provider communications and collaboration within population health management programs. Merely connecting providers to the Internet enables healthcare professionals to access information, search databases, communicate with peers, pursue continuing education, retrieve software and images, obtain prescribing drug information, and access statistical data (Burnham 1996; Satya-Murti 1993; Cohen and Strawn 1996; Robishaw and Roth 1994). There is also potential for follow-up education, continuing education (Sanders et al. 1995), and expanded access to services such as electronic mail and sophisticated medical information not traditionally available outside of academic medical centers (McGowan et al. 1995; Coggan and Crandall 1995). These education and information services can be tailored to fit the population health management approach being applied with greater potential benefits to involved participants and providers.

Personal Data Assistants (PDAs)

Personal data (or digital) assistants (PDAs)—also know as handheld computers, handheld devices, palms, or Palm Pilots™—are gaining popularity in both clinical and nonclinical settings. These small, handheld, functionally flexible, customizable, open-platform computers are increasingly being used at the point of patient care. Inherently portable, they retain the functionality of Internet connectivity and linkages to other computer networks, even when wireless.

Numerous and varied uses for PDAs in population health management exist. Their portability facilitates physician use at patients' bedsides, as well as care managers' use in home visits or remote patient monitoring. Physicians can use PDAs for day-to-day patient care operations such as communicating with peers and consults, researching medical and drug information, tracking patients, writing prescriptions, checking laboratory and other test results, ordering tests, charting patient data, coding, billing, and writing progress notes. Personal and workflow organization functions such as an address book and date book also permit ongoing patient management. It is currently estimated that 15 to 20 percent of physicians own Palm Pilots™ or their functional equivalents (W. R. Hambrecht and Company 2000), and this number is increasing rapidly.

The potential for PDAs to improve care and performance in population health management programs is immense. Software applications for PDAs are continuously being developed both through dedicated vendors and individual enthusiasts. Both physician-driven and care-manager-driven applications can help to improve patient monitoring and population health management processes. Such an IT tool, through its flexibility and portability, facilitates better management, both remotely and in person, of many different population groups by a wide variety of providers.

Drug Delivery Devices

The pharmaceutical industry offers another source of IT tools with tremendous potential to affect population health management approaches. As one example, devices to improve patient adherence and compliance with prescription drug regimens show considerable promise.

For patients who forget to take their medications, or those with regimens that require them to take pills at certain intervals, specially designed pill bottles incorporate alarm reminders. These pill bottles contain microchips that record when the bottle is opened and then sound an alarm when too much time has passed. Alarms are not reset until the pill bottle is opened. Of course, there is no guarantee that merely opening a bottle means a patient will take a pill. However, as long as the bottles are kept in a place where patients can hear the alarms, the reminder system has the potential to improve compliance in most medication management situations.

"Talking" pill bottles are another recent innovation to help improve patient compliance with medication management. Evidence suggests that as many as 40 percent of patients receiving prescriptions do not completely understand either the circumstances under which they should be taking the medication or the warnings associated with the prescription. Specially developed labels that are compatible with a device called ScripTalk can now be printed at major pharmacies . Estimated to cost about $200, ScripTalk is a handheld device containing a microchip that "reads" prescription drug labels aloud. For individuals who have trouble seeing or reading, this device improves their understanding of their medications. The device also helps patients who have multiple medications or who live in households with others who take prescription medications. The verbal directions can help ensure that they take the correct medication at the correct dosage.

Use of the Internet

Another form of information technology, the Internet, offers tremendous potential for population health management. The Internet has already proved immensely valuable as a health education tool, providing access to countless pages of health-related information. New web sites are regularly being developed to provide information about health and wellness to consumers and providers alike. Most health services organizations have also developed an institutional web sites for health-oriented content, as well as links to existing health and wellness information elsewhere on the Web.

Population health management programs can capitalize on the existence of this health education information by helping to sort through and organize the quantity of data available. However, the quality and credibility of healthcare information on the Internet is of concern to many individuals (Warson 1997). This concern has been recognized, and the not-for-profit organization URAC, formerly the American Accreditation Health Care Commission, recently released a list of accreditation standards for health sites on-line. This accreditation process is part of the effort to help consumers assess available health information, and to provide a means for users to report misinformation, privacy violations, and similar complaints. The over 50 criteria for sites to meet will enable them to receive the URAC seal of approval on their web sites. As of February 2002, 13 sites had received this seal of approval, including sites from WebMD, WellMed, IntelliHealth, the Health Insurance Association of America (HIAA), Healthwise, and Healthyroads (URAC 2002).

By distilling information into content appropriate for individuals or targeted groups, population health management programs can focus educational messages for their audiences. Mass customization is possible through the application of various algorithms that sort health information based on disease or health assessment criteria. In this way, individual participants can receive health education messages appropriate for their individual conditions. Furthermore, such messages can even be timed and directed to individuals at various intervals. If assessments such as readiness and willingness to change behaviors are included in a health management program, messages can be tailored based on the stage of an individual participant's readiness to hear about specific health intervention and behavior change options.

The Internet also provides a vehicle for population health management itself by virtue of its reach and flexibility. Health management programs that rely upon health assessment algorithms can use web-based technologies to develop dynamic health assessment approaches (as briefly described in the discussion of computer-driven algorithms). This capability allows the assessment process to be mass customized, tailored to the individual respondent while still maintaining a focus on the targeted population. Additional assessment modules can be incorporated into a general health assessment process or educational intervention, depending on respondent answers to individual questions or groups of questions. For example, a participant completing an assessment about health behaviors such as exercise and eating habits may answer a question about alcohol use that triggers further assessment about potential for alcohol and substance abuse. Alternatively, answering a question admitting to smoking will trigger a question about whether the individual would consider quitting, and so forth. While the previous scenarios are possible in the absence of the Internet, the use of web-based technology enhances the ability to link assessment modules and interweave questions based on respondent answers.

Another opportunity presented by the Internet is the ability to remotely monitor participants' health and clinical measurements in a form of telemedicine. As described above, devices have been developed that permit patients to check and record blood pressures, weights, blood sugars, and other measures using Internet technologies. Using such approaches, remote care managers can monitor patients' health status in real time. Furthermore, by incorporating an alert system such as electronic red flags on computer monitors or automatic pages, care managers can immediately react to readings that raise concern.

In his discussion of web-based disease management, Joch (2000) cites several promising new capabilities provided by the Internet including:

- technical flexibility that enables users to customize programs and add features;
- shorter implementation cycles resulting in system launches in as few as four months;
- better communications, including both business-to-business and physician-to-patient;
- patient empowerment providing patients with access to information relevant to their individual conditions; and
- the capability of the Web to deliver advice and recommendations impartially and bluntly ("tough love").

Many business have clearly taken advantage of these features to develop population health management capabilities, and, according to a survey in *Healthcare Informatics' 2000 Resource Guide*, at least 183 companies reportedly provide disease management software solutions alone (Joch 2000). Products such as password-protected applications that enable electronic prescribing, on-line medical chart applications, and additional pharmaceutical services that permit monitoring of chronic disease patients are among those offered by on-line disease management companies (Gomaa 2000).

The Internet also greatly enhances communication. Health management programs can take advantage of web-enabled interventions such as chat rooms with providers, support groups for individuals suffering from the same disease or condition, or instant messaging between care managers. Participants can be given electronic mail addresses to facilitate their communications with physicians and care managers who are helping them in the health management program. Web-based forms for patients can provide health, activity, or attitude information to care managers. Furthermore, interventions can be developed to promote better health and health management through the use of such communication technologies.

One health management strategy used the Internet to provide a behavioral weight loss program and compared results to those of a traditional behavioral therapy program. Participants who received the web-based program had a sequence of 24 behavioral lessons delivered weekly by e-mail, submitted self-monitoring diaries weekly to receive individualized feedback from a therapist via e-mail, and had access to an on-line bulletin board. Program results showed participants in the Internet-enhanced program lost more weight and were more likely to achieve their five-percent weight loss goal than participants in the standard education group (Tate et al. 2001).

The Internet can also be a powerful tool for coordination. Health management programs can take advantage of web-based technologies to monitor and track program participants. Coordination and communications among care managers is facilitated on the Web through communication tools such as e-mail, chat rooms, or even streaming video. Providers can coordinate among themselves as well as with care managers by having shared access to patient records, progress notes, and other data available on secure web sites. Web-based forms permit automatic faxes to primary care physicians or specialists involved in the management of individual patients. This enhanced coordination will only improve patient health and well-being through increased program participation by care providers. (See 14.3 "Web-based Tools" at www.ache.org/pubs/mcalearney/start.cfm.)

Security, Confidentiality, and Privacy

Considering IT as well as Internet use in healthcare obviously raises the issues of information security, privacy, and confidentiality. Information *security* refers to the protection of information from unauthorized access and can involve different mechanisms. Data encryption helps secure electronic data flow, and encryption-key access restricts access to only those authorized to view the data. Authorization is managed by authentication mechanisms including passwords, digital certificates, digital signatures, biometrics, and smart cards. Additional data security measures can include adequate backup of data, housing data in a secure environment (safe from theft, fire, flood; adequate air conditioning), and protecting information systems with firewalls. Security mechanisms help prevent unauthorized access to information and ensure the integrity of data contained in information systems.

Privacy of information involves the control of information access as dictated by the owner of or the subject of the information. In healthcare, privacy typically refers to the right of individual patients to control access to their own medical data. Security and privacy are complementary concepts, but it is possible for information to be secure, yet for violations of privacy to occur.

The issue of *confidentiality* of information is also critically important in healthcare. Confidentiality involves the element of trust and builds upon the concepts of security and privacy. In a healthcare setting, an individual patient may authorize access to his or her medical record in a secure environment, but give that authorization with the understanding that the medical information will not be shared with unauthorized personnel. Confidentiality represents the duty of the party trusted with the information to prevent further disclosure of that information.

All three issues have gained increased attention with recent legislation passed to address healthcare information. Specifically, the Health Insurance Portability and Accountability Act (HIPAA) of 1996 dictated how healthcare information must be stored, transmitted, and managed by healthcare organizations. Final rules to guide information management in healthcare and enforcement of those rules are the responsibility of the Department of Health and Human Services.

HIPAA legislation includes a variety of regulations addressing health-care information, including imposing standards for healthcare information exchange and for information security. Regulations addressing privacy and confidentiality of healthcare information as well as the rights of individual consumers to access their medical information have also been imposed.

In a population health management program environment, these issues are of considerable concern. One major issue affecting population health management programs is the security of electronic mail communications. Unless encoding and decoding of messages is included in an electronic mail program, sending e-mail is similar to sending a postcard through the mail. Programs that rely on e-mail for communications should not transmit sensitive or confidential information, nor should patient records or raw data be sent via electronic mail.

Another concern relevant to health management programs is the use of the legacy systems of different healthcare organizations. While the information contained in legacy systems is often critical for program purposes, most systems were not designed with the capabilities necessary for optimal information security. Relying on individual programmers or care managers to access clinical and financial information needed for health management program purposes requires a level of trust for both types of personnel. When it is not possible to impose authentication mechanisms or other security measures, programs face the added responsibility of training their employees to use sensitive healthcare information carefully and appropriately at all times.

Program use of the Internet raises a number of security issues that need to be continually addressed. Information can leak out of systems by way of theft by hackers, while unwanted information can also be introduced through viruses, worms, and so forth. Even good encryption is of limited protection because it only protects data in transit. To provide added protection, firewalls are very useful. By using a combination of routers and an application gateway, a firewall serves as an electronic drawbridge restricting access to unauthorized traffic. Including additional security measures such as authentication mechanisms can help ensure that sensitive healthcare information is kept as secure as possible.

Management Issues

The use of information technologies in population health management is also associated with a variety of management issues. Among these are considerations about resource requirements, physician involvement with technology, and training and implementation for selected information technologies.

Resource Requirements

Regardless of what information technologies are selected to improve the potential reach of population health management programs, resources will be required to incorporate such technologies. These resource requirements may range from relatively simple investment decisions such as the purchase of handheld devices to support care managers, to major capital investments.

Programs must consider resource requirements at the time of program design to ensure that appropriate resources are allocated. For programs that will rely heavily on Internet capabilities and web-based technologies, the issues of connectivity, bandwidth, and security may be paramount. Alternatively, programs choosing to rely more on existing legacy information systems may need less investment in new IT but a heavier commitment to data collection and analysis resources. More reliance on paper-based processes can involve a greater need for physical space and secure storage facilities. In contrast, moving to a paperless program format will entail increased attention to electronic security issues such as information access and medical record confidentiality. Additional investment may be necessary for programs that choose to incorporate new IT options such as remote clinical monitoring and other telemedicine activities. Considering these opportunities up front will help program designers develop realistic projections for budgetary requirements and associated institutional IT needs.

For program vendors reliant upon healthcare institutions to provide information about program participants in forms such as claims data, pharmacy data, or health surveys, contract discussions should also include consideration about the availability, accessibility, and reliability of required data. Contingency plans should be in place for when data are found to be missing or inaccurate.

Managers initiating population health management programs should be aware of the potential demands of these programs whether they are built in-house or outsourced. At the least, population health management programs will typically require a substantial investment in computer resources and will most likely benefit from speedy and reliable connectivity to the Internet. The more programs are able and willing to incorporate data from existing information systems, the greater the potential resource demands for management information systems support services such as queries, programming, or data translation. To the extent that it is possible to consider such demands up front, planning for program resource allocation, both financial and human, may be more accurate.

Physician Involvement

Another management issue related to the use of IT in population health management programs is the level of physician involvement expected. Many programs will rely on physicians who are not dedicated employees of the health management program, so it is important to consider both physician incentives to participate in the program and to comply with IT use requirements. Even physicians who are dedicated to the program in theory may find it difficult in practice to commit required time and resources. For programs that rely heavily on both physician involvement and sophisticated use of IT, it is especially important to include a training component in program roll-out. Developing user-friendly solutions that encourage physicians to participate and realize benefits from access to IT and to the program overall will be beneficial to all involved.

Limitations surrounding physician use of IT can range from inadequate systems and resources to a lack of interest or desire to participate. When resources are a constraint, management should consider the best interests of both patients and the program when making additional resource allocation decisions. It is possible that a simple investment, such as in a facsimile machine for a medical office, will permit willing physicians to participate. More serious limitations arise from physicians who are uncomfortable with IT. Physicians who wish to support patients in their health management goals but who do not choose to learn the technology will require either special training or specialized work-arounds to accommodate their participation. Additional training may also be necessary for office staff and other clinical personnel who are involved with caring for health management program patients.

Training and Implementation

Implementation issues for a population health management program that includes IT must take into account both the variety of information technologies and the range of personnel involved. Depending on the nature of the program and its components, the variability of each of these factors can be great.

Incorporating new and different types of IT into a population health management program will require training about how to use the IT. Training for care managers should be inclusive and introduce all types of IT that will be used by patients, providers, or the care managers themselves. Care managers should also be included in any technology development discussions to allow them to provide their perspective about how programs can be enhanced with technology. Incorporation of computer-based algorithms, for example, should proceed with clinician users and computer programmers working side by side to develop feasible and usable IT solutions. Similarly, inclusion of remote monitoring devices such as electronic scales or blood pressure cuffs in programs should be accompanied by both care manager and patient training to ensure that participants understand what to do, when to do it, and what to do if it does not work as expected.

Information technology training should be developed and tailored to respond to the needs of all trainees. Language differences, cultural sensitivities, literacy levels, differences in professional training, and levels of comfort with IT must all be addressed to successfully implement a program that relies upon IT. Trainers should leave participants with information regarding problem resolution or future training needs they may encounter. Furthermore, while health management programs may be able to operate in a paperless environment, regulations concerning documentation of patient contacts often still require paper reports. Clarifying expectations and requirements for documentation up front will ensure implementation and operation of health management programs proceed with as few problems as possible.

Additional implementation issues surrounding the use of IT in health management programs include factors such as space, human resources, and expectations about program communications. Space may be less of an issue for programs such as demand management services that rely largely on telephonic contacts, and some programs may contract with telephone banks for dedicated calling services. However, for programs that decide not to outsource call services, decisions about space allocation for IT and considerations such as privacy for patient telephone calls are very important.

Human resources issues related to the use of IT may range from realistically presenting IT-based job requirements to ensuring that clinicians hired can communicate effectively and confidently with IT personnel regarding their needs and concerns. Appropriate employee evaluation processes must be in place to ensure that personnel consistently and effectively use required IT. Outcomes assessment processes may include components such as patient satisfaction with IT or with the program, making it important for all employees to be committed to excellent service.

Finally, for programs that rely heavily on remote patient management for program activities, expectations about frequency, types, and consistency of communications with program personnel should be set forth. Patients and physicians may not be as comfortable with remote management as care managers, so care managers must make sure that client expectations are appropriately managed.

Conclusion

This chapter has presented a discussion of both the promise and pitfalls of using information technology in population health management. From telemedicine to handheld devices, the potential of many IT applications to improve the consistency, reach, and effectiveness of population health management interventions is great. However, concerns about information security and confidentiality, as well as management concerns about resource requirements, training, and IT implementation, should all be taken into consideration.

REFERENCES

Balas, E. A., F. Jaffrey, G. J. Kuperman, S. A. Boren, G. D. Brown, F. Pinciroli, and J. A. Mitchell. 1997. "Electronic Communication with Patients. Evaluation of Distance Medicine Technology." *Journal of the American Medical Association* 278 (2): 152–59.

Burnham, J. 1996. "Medical Information on the Internet." *Alabama Medicine* 65 (8–10): 9–13.

Burstein, J. L., M. C. Henry, J. Alicandro, D. Gentile, H. C. Thode, Jr., and J. E. Hollander. 1996. "Outcome of Patients who Refused Out-of-Hospital Medical Assistance." *American Journal of Emergency Medicine* 14 (1): 23–26.

Chande, V. T., N. Wyss, and V. Exum. 1996. "Educational Interventions to Alter Pediatric Department Utilization Patterns." *Archives of Pediatrics and Adolescent Medicine* 15(5): 525–28.

Coggan, J. M., and L. A. Crandall, L. A. 1995. "Expanding Rural Primary Care Training by Employing Information Technologies: The Need for Participation by Medical Reference Librarians." *Medical Reference Services Quarterly* 14 (1): 9–16.

Cohen, J. L., and E. L. Strawn. 1996. "Telemedicine in the '90s." *Journal of the Florida Medical Association* 83 (9): 631–33.

Davis, S. 1996. *Future Perfect*. Reading, MA: Addison-Wesley Publishing Company, Inc.

Derlet, R. W., D. Kinser, L. Ray, B. Hamilton, and J. McKenzie. 1995. "Prospective Identification and Triage of Nonemergency Patients Out of an Emergency Department: A 5-year Study." *Annals of Emergency Medicine* 25 (2): 215–23.

Gomaa, W. 2000. "Managing Expectations of Online Disease Management Programs." *Healthcare PR & Marketing News* 9 (5): 1–3.

Grigsby, J., M. M. Kaehny, E. J. Sandbert, R. E. Schlenker, and P. W. Shaughnessy. 1995. "Effects and Effectiveness of Telemedicine" *Health Care Financing Review* 17 (1): 27–34.

Grigsby, J., and J. H. Sanders. 1998. "Telemedicine: Where It Is and Where It's Going." *Annals of Internal Medicine* 129 (2): 123–27.

itmWeb. 2002. "MIS Spending Benchmarks." [On-line information; accessed 8/8/02.] http://www.itmweb.com/blbenchbgt.htm.

Joch, A. 2000. "Can the Web Save Disease Management?" *Healthcare Informatics* (March). [On-line article; retrieved 6/7/02.] http://www.healthcare-informatics.com/issues/2000/03_00/cover.htm.

McGowan, J., J. Evans, and K. Michl. 1995. "Networking a Need: A Cost-effective Approach to Statewide Health Information Delivery." *Proceedings of the 18th Annual Symposium on Computer Applications in Medical Care*. Philadelphia, PA: Hanley & Belfus, Inc.

McGrory, B. J, A. A. Shinar, A. A. Freiberg, and W. H. Harris. 1997. "Enhancement of the Value of Hip Questionnaires by Telephone Follow-up Evaluation." *Journal of Arthroplasty* 12 (3): 340–43.

Marcus, A. C., and L. A. Crane. 1998. "A Review of Cervical Cancer Screening Intervention Research: Implications for Public Health Programs and Future Research." *Preventive Medicine* 27 (1): 13–31.

McAlearney, A. S. 2002. "Population Health Management in Theory and Practice." In *Advances in Health Care Management* (Volume 3), edited by G. T. Savage, J. Blair, and M. Fottler. New York: JAI Press/Elsevier Science Ltd.

Moore, G. B., B. E. Reynolds, and D. A. Ray. 1995. "Information Architects: Data by Design." *HMO Magazine* 36 (3): 29–31, 34–35.

Nash, I. S. 2000. "Dynamic Assessment in Disease Management." *Disease Management and Health Outcomes* 8 (3): 139–46.

Patton, K., J. Meyers, and B. E. Lewis. 1997. "Enhancement of Compliance Among Patients with Hypertension." *American Journal of Managed Care* 3 (11): 1693–98.

Perednia, D. A., and A. Allen. 1995. "Telemedicine Technology and Clinical Applications." *Journal of the American Medical Association* 273 (6): 483–88.

"Predict Utilization and Get More Bang for Your DM Dollars." 1998. *Healthcare Demand and Disease Management* 4 (9): 141–43.

Reese, R. G., and R. Majzun. 2000. "Information Systems and Electronic Commerce for Provider Systems in Managed Health Care." In *The Managed Care Handbook*, 4th ed., edited by P. Kongstvedt. Gaithersburg, MD: Aspen Publishers.

Robishaw, S. M., and B. G. Roth. 1994. "Grateful Med-Loansome Doc Outreach Project in Central Pennsylvania." *Bulletin of the Medical Library Association* 82 (2): 206–13.

Rolnick, S. J., D. Klevan, L. Cherney, and H. A. Lando. 1997. "Nicotine Replacement Therapy in a Group Model HMO" *HMO Practice* 11 (1): 34–37.

Sanders, J., P. Brucker, and M. D. Miller. 1995. "Using Telemedicine for Continuing Education for Rural Physicians." *Academic Medicine* 70 (5): 457.

Satya-Murti, S. 1993. "A Core Electronic Medical Library in a Rural Setting: Update." *Kansas Medicine* 94 (10): 264–67.

Simon, J. A., S. N. Solkowitz, T. P. Carmody, and W. S. Browner. "Smoking Cessation After Surgery. A Randomized Trial." *Archives of Internal Medicine* 157 (12): 1371–76.

Tate, D. F., R. R. Wing, and R. A. Winett. 2001. "Using Internet Technology to Deliver a Behavioral Weight Loss Program." *Journal of the American Medical Association* 285 (9): 1172–77.

URAC. 2002. "Health Web Site Accreditation." Washington, DC: URAC. [On-line information; retrieved 2/24/02.] http://websiteaccreditation.urac.org.

Warson, A. 1997. "Care from a Distance. Web Sites, Video, E-mail Have Growing Treatment Roles." *Modern Healthcare* 27 (14): 132, 134.

W. R. Hambrecht and Company. 2000. "The Cure Is In Hand." [On-line article; accessed 8/8/02.] http://www.medicalwindows.com/research/TheCure.pdf.

CHAPTER

15

CONCLUSION: LEVERAGING OPPORTUNITIES IN POPULATION HEALTH MANAGEMENT

This book was written to provide an overview of population health management strategies that can be effectively implemented for defined populations. Implementation of such strategies, however, often poses a major challenge for managers and healthcare practitioners. As a conclusion to this book, this chapter describes ten critical considerations for practitioners interested in pursuing population health management strategies. Finally, five areas of consideration are presented for health services researchers committed to the concepts of population health management. Keeping in mind these critical areas can help program designers, developers, and evaluators best leverage the opportunities created by population health management strategies.

Critical Considerations for Managers and Healthcare Practitioners

Applying a population health management strategy should be an option for most defined populations. For the managers, practitioners, and policy makers responsible for the individual members of those populations, population health management strategies can improve health and health outcomes while lowering medical care costs. This book has presented a number of strategies and concepts designed to promote population health improvements. However, achieving success with any strategy relies on multiple factors. Ten of these critical considerations for managers and healthcare practitioners follow:

1. Clarify population definition
2. Identify resource constraints for the program
3. Establish program goals and desired outcomes
4. Maintain a consumer focus
5. Develop and enhance relationships with providers
6. Leverage the value of information technologies
7. Work to align financial incentives

8. Concentrate on program implementation
9. Focus on quality improvement
10. Strive for greater integration

Clarify Population Definition

As described in Chapter 3, defining the target population for a population health management strategy is critical. Not only does the definition of the population delimit the individuals to be served, but it also establishes the parameters for a health management strategy. Targeting an elderly population will present different health management challenges than will targeting a younger, employed population. An employed population consisting of lower-income women such as that hired by a nursing home will have different health needs than a higher-income population working for an engineering firm. Clarifying this definition of population up front is one of the first steps in developing an effective population health management program to serve the needs of the individuals targeted.

Identify Resource Constraints

Another initial step in developing a population health management program is the identification of any resource constraints. While resources are limited in any environment, determining the amount of resources available and any constraints on those resources is crucial to program development. For example, community health departments may have resources available to provide primary prevention services such as immunizations for their target population, but their resources for tertiary prevention services may be limited at best. Establishing what resources are available for a given program and then evaluating whether, and to what extent, those resources are constrained, focuses program design activities and permits establishment of achievable program goals.

Establish Program Goals and Desired Outcomes

Both population definition and the identification of resource constraints are clearly linked to some determination of program goals. Coming to agreement about desired goals and objectives for a health management program helps to appropriately focus program design. Taking into consideration opportunities for or barriers to program development based on population definition and resource constraints enables program designers to specify reasonable goals and desired outcomes and then match the population health management strategy to these goals. Specifying reasonable program outcomes up front permits programs to achieve success through targeted program development and effective program implementation.

Maintain Consumer Focus

Whether individual participants in a health management program are identified as members, patients, persons, or consumers, maintaining a focus on these individuals is another key to program success. Population health management strategies are, by definition, focused on the health and medical care needs of populations. However, providing services and care to these populations occurs on an individual basis. While mass communication strategies such as mailings, newsletters, or web pages may be available, the interaction between the individual consumer and the population health management program is a crucial interface. Consumers who do not feel their questions are answered well or who feel they are treated poorly by a provider or institution are likely to report dissatisfaction with their experience in the health management program and share this negative experience with others. By focusing on consumer needs and perceptions at the multiple interaction points, a program is more likely to meet those needs and satisfy its consumers. Furthermore, by maintaining a focus on consumers and consumer health, the goals of health improvement and consumer wellness will most likely be achieved.

Develop and Enhance Provider Relationships

From the perspective of many population health management programs, a second major consumer is the provider. Particularly for those participating providers who are not officially affiliated with a population health management program, service to these individuals is an area of vital program focus. Communications about program expectations must be stated clearly to minimize the possibility of misunderstandings. Good communication also keeps program goals aligned with provider goals and expectations. For physician providers especially, any program-initiated follow-up with patients should be coordinated with participating physician involvement. Because most population health management programs cannot succeed without a solid commitment from physician providers, maximizing provider satisfaction with the program is a critical consideration.

Leverage the Value of Information Technologies

As described in Chapter 14, the opportunities presented by information technologies can be invaluable for population health management programs. To take advantage of such opportunities, however, program designers must ensure that programs commit a sufficient level of resources to investment in appropriate information technologies. While many established health services organizations have not yet positioned themselves on the cutting edge of information systems and information technologies, development of a population health management strategy can present an opportunity to explore this position. Possibilities for utilizing information technologies to identify program participants, screen them, assess health risk status, target individuals for interventions, tailor interventions, and maintain ongoing communications are abundant in the population health management field. Incorporating information technology can maximize the potential for program success.

Work To Align Financial Incentives

In the health services sector as in any other industry, the alignment of financial incentives to encourage appropriate behavior is important. Institutions and even physician providers may knowingly or unknowingly work at cross purposes because of their level of assumed financial risk and responsibilities towards patients. Carrying financial risk for a population of individuals should create appropriate incentives for health management within that population. The challenge for population health management strategies, however, is to clarify the perspective of the program to determine where incentives lie and attempt to develop a program that is consistent with the goals of the payers and providers involved. Maintaining a focus on consumers helps to ensure that improvements in health and wellness are primary program goals. However, the financial objectives of providers and payers are important as well. Program developers must strive to design a strategy that recognizes where financial risk has been delegated and works to encourage health management activities along those risk lines.

Concentrate on Program Implementation

Even with impeccable design, population health management program success depends on strong implementation. Managers and healthcare practitioners must attempt to minimize implementation barriers as programs are initiated and operate. In fact, each of the other critical considerations already described here may involve implementation challenges. While it is important to define a population to be served, an implementation step must involve identifying individual members of that population and encouraging such individuals to participate. Resource requirements must clearly consider both program implementation and operations, and the establishment of program goals may be constrained by implementation issues as they affect the reasonableness of program outcomes expected for the defined population. The selection of information technologies will also affect program implementation and progress. Finally, relationships with providers will affect the extent to which a population health management program can suggest and encourage changes in standard provider behavior to improve health and wellness for the population targeted. Concentrating on the multiple facets of program implementation increases the likelihood that population health management programs achieve their goals and desired outcomes.

Quality Improvement Focus

Another important focus for population health management programs is on quality improvement or Continuous Quality Improvement (CQI). Whether a formal, institutionalized program of CQI or a less formal program structure of assessment, revision, and reassessment in a modified approach to the plan-do-check-act cycle, it is important to consider quality improvement in any population health management program. As discussed, a focus on program goals and outcomes is critical to define and achieve program success. Building a quality improvement framework into a population health management program necessarily involves an evaluative component that permits measurement of defined goals and outcomes. Assessment or evaluation of intermediate program outcomes enables managers and practitioners to modify program components if the program is progressing differently than expected. Operational modifications and program enhancements in the context of quality improvement can then help programs to achieve their goals within the budget constraints and defined parameters. Focusing on quality improvement within a health management program encourages all participants to work together to achieve both intermediate and ultimate program outcomes such as lower costs, better quality of healthcare, and improved health.

Strive for Greater Integration

Striving for greater integration is the tenth critical consideration for population health management programs. As discussed in Chapter 10, an integrated population health management strategy is consistent with the goals of improved health and wellness in all population health management strategies. However, even when a fully integrated model cannot be developed, programs can still realize benefits from greater levels of integration. Integrated information systems permit more reliable identification, monitoring, and assessment of individuals targeted for program participation. Similarly, integration of clinical goals by means of clear communication and coordination between and among providers benefits all patients. Integrated communications can help reduce consumer confusion about mixed or even contradictory health messages. Furthermore, an integrated program reporting function presents a picture of program progress towards goals and outcomes that is comprehensive and appropriate for multiple audiences. Ideally, striving for greater integration fosters a better appreciation for individual health and wellness in the context of population health.

Areas of Focus for Health Services Researchers

Population health management strategies are, by design, very outcomes-oriented. Health services researchers and other academics can make valuable contributions to the design, development, and evaluation of each of the population health management strategies discussed in this text. In practice, five key areas of population health management are particularly congruent with the expertise of many health services researchers:

1. Focus on outcomes
2. Data and information management
3. Apply theory and research evidence to program development

4.   Share program research results
5.   Broaden perspective of population health management programs

Focus on Outcomes

The importance of outcomes measurement and monitoring in population health management cannot be overemphasized. Health services researchers have the ability to contribute substantially to both program development and results by helping designers consider the implications of focusing on particular program outcomes.

First, selection of program outcomes is necessarily linked to the definition of the population served. An employed population may have different program outcome goals than that of a population of Medicare beneficiaries covered by a particular insurance plan. Defining the population appropriately and then developing metrics to tie desired outcomes and goals to that population are useful contributions of health services researchers. Researchers can establish baseline measurements of health indices and other population information relevant in program outcome assessment. In addition, ongoing monitoring and feedback about program progress and results are similarly measurement-intensive processes that can be improved by partnership with trained program evaluators.

Including researchers in the design stage of population health management programs facilitates later program evaluation in multiple ways. Health services researcher expertise in the areas of outcomes research and program evaluation can help with establishment of program goals and outcomes that are both reasonable and measurable. Because hypotheses and anticipated outcomes are best specified at the outset, the early involvement of health services research can help ensure that evaluations are both objective and inclusive.

In addition to final outcome measures, interim measures to monitor program progress should also be specified. Researchers can help with development of interim outcome measures as well as process measures or other measures of program success. Evaluation midpoints can be assessed and information provided to program developers to guide any program adjustments that might be appropriate. As an example, information about insufficient ability to reach individual members in a target population can be used to modify participant recruitment strategies and encourage program involvement by both patient members and providers. Including health services researchers who consider outcomes measurement and improvement in program design and development can help population health management programs more reliably and definitively reach program goals.

Data and Information Management

Directly related to a focus on outcomes is an appreciation for the expertise health services researchers typically have in data and information management. While there are certainly many types of academic specialists, researchers who work with different types of health services data can provide invaluable advice to population health management programs. From monitoring data quality to ensuring appropriate data collection strategies to final data analyses, health services researchers can work as program partners in many ways.

Population health management strategies require the use of different types of personal, health, financial, and clinical data on an ongoing basis. As described in Chapter 4, participants must be identified—usually through existing databases or some type of screening questionnaire—before finely tuned targeting for program participation can begin. Researchers with expertise in health surveys or risk screening tools can help program developers ask appropriate questions of the target population. Experts in survey research and program evaluation can also provide ongoing support and make suggestions about validated survey tools or about how to validate proposed surveys for use in different population health management programs.

Apply Theory and Research Evidence to Program Development

Health services researchers and academics also add value to population health management strategies by incorporating theory and research evidence into programs. Many population health management programs have theoretical bases and the appropriate application of these theories can help programs succeed. Chapter 10 has included discussion of some of these important applications. In addition, recognition of the tenets of learning theory and psychology can assist with the development of targeted and effective lifestyle management programs. Similarly, specialists in health behavior change can help program developers design health management strategies that are appropriate for different defined populations.

Organizational theories are applicable in the areas of change management as employers, payers, and health services organizations are challenged to develop a culture in which the concepts of population health management and health improvement are the norm. Similarly, theories related to diffusion of innovation can help as organizations struggle to incorporate information technologies into population health management programs and their broader organizations. Theoretical work related to the importance of teams in organizations is especially useful when applied in the context of population health management programs reliant on multidisciplinary teams of physician providers and other caregivers.

Moving beyond theory, academic researchers can serve as very effective conduits as they translate relevant research findings into practice. New evidence about treatment methodologies, intervention effectiveness and cost-effectiveness, and clinical care delivery can be incorporated in many population health management strategies. Health services researchers may also be able to provide a broad research perspective that helps programs focus on opportunities for integration of different health and care management strategies. Considerations about expanding program offerings to move towards an integrated population health management strategy can have benefits for patients, practitioners, and researchers alike.

Finally, specialized knowledge about different population groups is invaluable. Working with gerontologists and geriatricians who have expertise with the elderly can be effective in program development when strategies must be tailored to an older population. Similarly, researchers who have studied particular diseases or treatment approaches can translate appropriate findings into clinical practice in the context of population health management programs. Clinicians and researchers who have analyzed population groups in different types of studies can offer ideas about appropriate population definition, stratification, and targeted interventions.

Share Program Research Results

Health services researchers are also well-positioned to evaluate population health management programs and share the results of such research, especially through publication. Whether publication occurs in peer-reviewed journals, trade journals, or trade magazines, dissemination of program results promotes the overall goals of improved population health. Sharing negative results as well can help other program developers avoid problems and pitfalls that have plagued unsuccessful programs. Opportunities also exist for researchers to broaden the reach of their findings by making contacts with policy makers and news media when appropriate. This wider dissemination of results in cases where population health management is truly making a difference in the health and wellness of a defined population extends opportunities for population health management programs and improves health for other populations.

Broaden Perspective of Population Health Management Programs

Health services researchers can also have an impact on broadening the perspective of population health management programs. Although individual programs may have a narrow focus and a narrowly defined population, program impact may be replicated in other settings.

Many population health management programs are limited in their focus because they have defined a target population and health improvement goals within an insured and reimbursed group of individuals. However, when population health management strategies successfully improve health and wellness and are demonstrated to save money in medical care expenses, extension of these strategies to other populations clearly makes sense. Hospitals working to provide coverage for their uninsured population can find value in applying relatively inexpensive lifestyle management or demand management strategies to support better self-care management and medical care utilization decisions. Similarly, providers may support extending disease management and catastrophic care management strategies to a broader population if such strategies indeed cost less and have equal or better health outcomes.

Health services researchers can encourage other potential program sponsors and policy makers to apply successful population health management principles and strategies to new settings and new populations. With a broader health policy perspective, researchers can speculate or model the possibilities of expanding population health management strategies to include and serve populations such as the uninsured, the underinsured, and the underserved.

Although finding payers to support the initial investment in such programs will be challenging, the opportunity to improve health and reduce longer-term medical care costs is undeniably appealing. It may be the role of federal, state, or local governments to support investment in and development of such initiatives. Health services researchers can provide both the financial and clinical justification for these commitments with carefully executed program evaluations and clearly presented research findings.

Taking advantage of the knowledge and expertise of health services researchers in different fields clearly offers multiple benefits for population health management programs. Lifestyle management and demand management programs will benefit from thoughtful application of theory as well as appropriate targeting of patients for interventions. Disease management and catastrophic care management programs can leverage current research findings to offer best practices in acute and rehabilitative care services for affected patients. Similar benefits will accrue to disability management programs and other strategies that strive towards greater integration of services across a continuum. Including researchers in program design, development, implementation, and evaluation is extremely valuable for population health management strategies hoping to improve patient health and wellness using the best evidence available.

Final Thoughts

As in any area of healthcare, opportunities in population health management are not stagnant. Medical care and health services research provide a steady flow of findings on which to base decisions about appropriate healthcare delivery. New research in genomics affects both targeting of individuals and delivery of interventions. New information technologies make many of the processes of population health management both more feasible and less expensive. Programs must be open to new possibilities and options for health and care management as they strive to improve care and service for their defined populations.

Strategies designed to improve population health and wellness are vitally important. This book has presented several strategies to foster health and quality of care improvements while managing costs. Health services organizations faced with the challenge of managing financial risk for defined populations must leverage opportunities to more efficiently and effectively serve such populations. Maintaining a focus on individual and patient needs within a population while supporting strategies to improve health and medical services along the continuum of care is the promise inherent in population health management.

INDEX

ABOUT THE AUTHOR

Ann Scheck McAlearney, Sc.D., is an Assistant Professor of Health Services Management and Policy at the Ohio State University. She holds bachelor's degrees in Biological Sciences and English from Stanford University, a master's degree in Biological Sciences from Stanford University, and a doctorate in Health Policy and Management from Harvard University. Professor McAlearney teaches courses in Health Services Organizational Management, Strategic Management and Program Development, and Leadership in Healthcare.

Dr. McAlearney's general research interests include outcomes research, population health management, information technology innovation, and healthcare leadership. Her publications cover issues such as access to care, satisfaction with care, disease management and population health management, information technology, cost-effectiveness of new technologies, and quality measurement. She is especially interested in how health services research findings are applied in healthcare organizations and how the reporting of healthcare outcomes and quality measures can be used to improve both care delivery and healthcare decision making by consumers.

Prior to returning to academics, Dr. McAlearney served as vice president for program development with Monsanto Health Solutions' VIHMS project, based in Los Angeles. In this role she directed the development of a web-based care management software product designed to integrate data and coordinate care for a Medicare risk population served by an integrated delivery system. She has also held positions and had consulting arrangements with organizations, including UniHealth, PacifiCare Health Systems, Merck & Co., Massachusetts General Hospital, Harvard School of Public Health, UCLA Medical Center, Arthur Young & Company, the Congressional Budget Office, and the World Health Organization.